"Steven Stern's *Needed Relationship and Psychoanalytic Healing* is an innovative and erudite work of scholarship and, perhaps more importantly, it is a leading-edged contribution to clinical psychoanalytic practice and education. Stern utilizes Louis Sander's developmental concept of progressive 'fittedness,' as a central organizing principle, and he systematically examines and illustrates the complex clinical implications of this paradigm. Focusing especially on the dialectics of understanding and relational engagement, and of conscious and unconscious participation, Stern advocates a holistic relational approach that uses but transcends theory in co-creating forms of engagement contoured to the uniquely evolving aims and needs of each patient. Compelling and rich clinical examples allow the reader to not only follow how Stern himself utilizes his multi-modelled pluralistic approach but more importantly, they allow readers to imagine how they themselves can make use of these conceptualizations to find creative and unique solutions to improving the quality of their understanding and engagement with patients. This book will be essential reading for students and sophisticated mental-health practitioners."—**Lewis Aron, Ph.D.**, Director, New York University Postdoctoral Program in Psychotherapy & Psychoanalysis.

"Culled from Stern's decades of intensive immersion in both the theory and the practice of analytic therapy, *Needed Relationship and Psychoanalytic Healing* explores, in richly satisfying detail, the nuances and subtleties of the moment-to-moment encounter between patient and therapist. It is a lovingly crafted, synergistic blend of elements that are at once self psychological, relational, existential, humanistic, empathic, present-focused, attachment-based, and systemic—a holistic view of the analytic relationship that appreciates both its simplicity and its complexity. Stern, clearly a brilliantly integrative scholar and an exquisitely gifted clinician, is able to hone in, with precision and finesse, on the very essence of the therapeutic process.

Ever mindful of avoiding dogma, Stern has masterfully found a way to tease out a number of 'organizing principles' specifically designed to provide the therapist with a broad-based conceptual—and contextual—framework for understanding both the patient's subjectivity and the ever-evolving intersubjective dynamic between patient and therapist—at the same time that this framework encourages the therapist not only to be mindful of all that is emerging at the 'points of emotional urgency' and in the 'moments of meeting' between patient and therapist but also to be attuned to the gradually unfolding and ever-evolving 'relational fittedness' between them. Chapter after chapter, we are gently reminded that, although we need theory to help guide us, it is important that we never allow it to get in the way of our ability to be present with our patients—so that we will have the freedom to find both them and 'us.'

Stern's book, a humane and accessible narrative that both inspires and is inspired, should be required reading for therapists of all levels." —**Martha Stark, MD**, Faculty, Harvard Medical School; Co-Director, Center for Psychoanalytic Studies; Faculty, Psychiatry Redefined.

"Steve Stern has given us a thorough interrogation of the central issues being debated in contemporary psychoanalysis today. His book demonstrates breadth and depth of scholarship at a level of detail that would take our collective breath away if it did not simultaneously breathe fresh new life into almost every psychoanalytic question ever asked. Stern lays out our current theoretical and technical conflicts using densely muscular prose that is at the same time finely chiseled in both style and content. And in his clinical vignettes, not only does each of his patients come achingly alive in her individuality and suffering, but so too does Steve Stern come alive as the struggling psychoanalyst. This book moves 21st century psychoanalytic discourse forward." —**Judith Guss Teicholz, Ph.D.**, Massachusetts Institute for Psychoanalysis.

"A unique characteristic of Stern's writing is that he absorbs, draws from, and integrates the best of so many analytic writers. I haven't seen anyone else do this so well. He tries for an integration of what he sees as the best of psychoanalysis, and then uses this integrative vision as the basis for his own original and valuable perspective on the psychoanalytic process and therapeutic action." —**James William Anderson, Ph.D.**, Northwestern University and the Chicago Institute for Psychoanalysis.

"Steven Stern has written an amazing book. *Needed Relationships and Psychoanalytic Healing* not only offers the sophisticated, psychoanalytically informed clinician a refreshing and integrating vision of the field, it provides at the same time a thorough-going education for the novice in the profession. If I had my way as an educator, I would insist that every psychoanalytic institute include in its training program for both the psychotherapist and the psychoanalyst-in-training an opportunity to study this book in full. I myself am teaching a course in psychoanalytic technique for the advanced candidates in psychoanalytic training at ICP, and Stern's book is the backbone of my syllabus." —**Estelle Shane, Ph.D.**, Founding member and training analyst, Institute for Contemporary Psychoanalysis, Los Angeles, CA.

Needed Relationships and Psychoanalytic Healing

Needed Relationships and Psychoanalytic Healing is both a personal analytic *credo* and a multidimensional approach to thinking about clinical interaction. The book's central theme is that of *analytic needed relationships*—the science and art of co-creating unique, evolving relational experiences fitted to each patient's implicit therapeutic aims and needs.

Steven Stern argues that, while we need psychoanalytic theories to "grow the receptors and processors" necessary to sense, understand, and connect with our patients, these often tend to frame the therapist's participation in terms of theoretical and technical categories rather than offering a more holistic view of the relationship in all of its human complexity. Stern believes that a new set of higher order constructs is needed to counteract this tendency. In addition to his own concept of needed relationships, he invokes principles from the work of renowned developmental researcher and theorist, Louis Sander: especially his concept of relational *fittedness.* Stern draws on the work of Freud, Bion, Winnicott, Kohut, and a broad spectrum of contemporary psychoanalytic authors, in fleshing out the therapeutic implications of Sander's (and Stern's own) vision. The result is a rich, humane, and accessible narrative.

Needed Relationships and Psychoanalytic Healing offers diverse clinical examples in which you will find Stern engaging with each of his patients in idiomatic, spontaneous ways as he attempts to contour interventions to the evolving analytic situation. This case material will inspire therapist-readers to feel freer to find their own creative voices and idioms of participation, as they seek to meet each patient within the psychoanalytic space. The book is intended for psychoanalysts and psychodynamic therapists at all levels of experience, including those in training.

Steven Stern, PsyD, is Clinical Associate Professor of Psychiatry at Maine Medical Center and Tufts University School of Medicine, faculty member at the Massachusetts Institute for Psychoanalysis, and a member of the International Council of the International Association of Psychoanalytic Self Psychology. He practices in Portland, Maine, with specializations in psychoanalysis, psychodynamic psychotherapy, couples therapy, and clinical supervision.

PSYCHOANALYSIS IN A NEW KEY BOOK SERIES

DONNEL STERN
Series Editor

When music is played in a new key, the melody does not change, but the notes that make up the composition do: change in the context of continuity, continuity that perseveres through change. Psychoanalysis in a New Key publishes books that share the aims psychoanalysts have always had, but that approach them differently. The books in the series are not expected to advance any particular theoretical agenda, although to this date most have been written by analysts from the Interpersonal and Relational orientations.

The most important contribution of a psychoanalytic book is the communication of something that nudges the reader's grasp of clinical theory and practice in an unexpected direction. Psychoanalysis in a New Key creates a deliberate focus on innovative and unsettling clinical thinking. Because that kind of thinking is encouraged by exploration of the sometimes surprising contributions to psychoanalysis of ideas and findings from other fields, Psychoanalysis in a New Key particularly encourages interdisciplinary studies. Books in the series have married psychoanalysis with dissociation, trauma theory, sociology, and criminology. The series is open to the consideration of studies examining the relationship between psychoanalysis and any other field—for instance, biology, literary and art criticism, philosophy, systems theory, anthropology, and political theory.

But innovation also takes place within the boundaries of psychoanalysis, and Psychoanalysis in a New Key therefore also presents work that reformulates thought and practice without leaving the precincts of the field. Books in the series focus, for example, on the significance of personal values in psychoanalytic practice, on the complex interrelationship between the analyst's clinical work and personal life, on the consequences for the clinical situation when patient and analyst are from different cultures, and on the need for psychoanalysts to accept the degree to which they knowingly satisfy their own wishes during treatment hours, often to the patient's detriment.

For a full list of all the titles in the Psychoanalysis in a New Key series, please visit the Routledge website.

Recent titles in the series

Vol. 33 *Needed Relationships and Psychoanalytic Healing: A Holistic Relational Perspective on the Therapeutic Process* Steven Stern

Vol. 32 *The Age of Perversion: Desire and Technology in Psychoanalysis and Culture* Danielle Knafo and Rocco Lo Bosco

Vol. 31 *Unknowable, Unspeakable and Unsprung: Psychoanalytic Perspectives on Truth, Scandal, Secrets and Lies* Edited by Jean Petrucelli and Sarah Schoen

Vol. 30 *Trauma and Countertrauma, Resilience and Counterresilience: Insights from Psychoanalysts and Trau ma Experts* Edited by Richard B. Gartner

Needed Relationships and Psychoanalytic Healing

A Holistic Relational Perspective on the Therapeutic Process

Steven Stern

Routledge
Taylor & Francis Group
LONDON AND NEW YORK

First published 2017
by Routledge
2 Park Square, Milton Park, Abingdon, Oxon OX14 4RN

and by Routledge
605 Third Avenue, New York, NY 10017

Routledge is an imprint of the Taylor & Francis Group, an informa business

British Library Cataloguing in Publication Data
A catalogue record for this book is available from the British Library

Library of Congress Cataloging in Publication Data
Names: Stern, Steven, 1948- author.
Title: Needed relationships and psychoanalytic healing : a holistic relational perspective on the therapeutic process/Steven Stern.Other titles: Psychoanalysis in a new key book series ; v. 33.
Description: Abingdon, Oxon ; New York, NY : Routledge, 2017. | Series: Psychoanalysis in a new key book series; volume 33 | Includes bibliographical references and index.
Identifiers: LCCN 2016040051| ISBN 9780415707879 (hardback : alk. paper) | ISBN 9780415707893 (pbk. : alk. paper) | ISBN 9781315268316 (e-book)
Subjects: | MESH: Psychoanalytic Therapy | Psychotherapeutic Processes | Interpersonal Relations | Unconscious (Psychology) | Transference (Psychology) | Holistic Health
Classification: LCC RC506 | NLM WM 460.6 | DDC 616.89/17—dc23
LC record available at https://lccn.loc.gov/2016040051

ISBN: 978-0-415-70787-9 (hbk)
ISBN: 978-0-415-70789-3 (pbk)
ISBN: 978-1-315-26831-6 (ebk)

Typeset in Times New Roman
by Swales & Willis Ltd, Exeter, Devon, UK

For Laura and Natalie

Contents

Preface

Some years back, my friend Steve Stern and I, grandly imagining ourselves the peacemakers in the ancient and endless psychoanalytic wars and schisms, imagined something we called our "common ground" project. Searching out the threads of agreement in the tangle of theories, institutes, journals, associations, pacifying old acrimonies and binding up old wounds, we would invent an inclusive conversation in our beloved profession. Beating theoretical swords into coffee hours, or even better, into dialogue over good wine, we would mend psychoanalysis for the present and future, presenting a more attractive field to potential candidates, a more usable and less technical form of treatment, and best of all, a psychoanalytic community in which we and our colleagues could live, learn, support each other, and grow old together. We would leave to the next generation a psychoanalysis less damaged by the traumatic cruelties of the past, and more ready to take on the challenges of the future.

The book you are about to read and enjoy resulted in part from these imaginings. We had not wished only for pluralism, modeled on even the most genuine acceptance of different cultures and religions. Inclusion, even in Buber's profound meaning of valorization of human dignity (important as this was to us), still left us with mere plurality, even the plurality of good things. We wanted something more. We sought for ideas and values that truly united us, that would make the timeworn disputes so secondary as to recede in the face of our compelling human concern. But I wandered off into ethics, and Steve was left to go on to think out the common ground, given all the enormous multiplicity, the non-dialogue and isolation, the continuing animosities of contemporary psychoanalysis. As I have followed him these last years, and read what he provides now, it seems to me he has followed two threads, intricately woven here, in his search for common ground, now articulated as his own psychoanalytic ground.

First, of course, comes clinical experience. His lived clinical experiences, in the plural, struggled with and reflected upon, have formed a body of experience. This book, full of stories both illustrating his complex ideas and leading us along his journey, shows how he allowed his patients to teach him. Instead of blaming them for their troubles, pathologizing them, instead of taking a *Besserwisser* (knowing better) attitude toward their protests and reproaches, he learns and questions, asking what many of the prominent contemporary theorists would say to this patient. Having already told us what he said or did, he then asks what we can generalize, within the long history of psychoanalysis and its contemporary conversations. How can we make sense of a way of working that he and many of us already use, what I informally call "bumbling along together," in search of emergent answers to Frieda Fromm-Reichmann's habitual question: "How can I help you?" In other words, what does this patient need from me that I cannot know in advance of the meeting or dialogue? What is the needed relationship?

Stern's formulation, much more elegant than my bumbling, brings out the second and most important theoretical emphasis on fittedness, for which he acknowledges his heavy indebtedness to Louis Sander, treasured pioneer in infant research, complexity thinking, and their usefulness in psychoanalysis. Inspiration to relationalists of many stripes, and to all psychoanalytic developmentalists, Sander, like Winnicott in his own idiom, taught us that the search for the other in nonlinear, relational time, begins wherever we begin and lasts as long as we last. Because one party to the search for relational fittedness always bears asymmetrical responsibility—the parent, the analyst, the teacher, the rabbi—we may forget that both are seeking and influencing. Disrupted by early or later trauma, haunted by traumatic residues across the generations, this search may turn demanding and difficult, leading analysts to speak of impasses and enactments. But we are always enacting the search for understanding, and its disruption, as this book reports. The patient seeks to fit us to his or her needs, "contouring," Stern calls it, while we seek to find the emotional and theoretical resources at every moment to meet the original and emergent needs of the suffering human being who seeks our care. Often, we resist this shaping by the patient, this stretching of our comfort zone, this challenging of our biases. Then we write and talk about defense and resistance, rarely referring to our own. When we can embrace the vulnerabilities this work demands of us, our patients and we may have the good fortune gradually to find and create the needed relationship, the needed fittedness.

I commend this book to its readers for a deeply thoughtful read.

Donna M. Orange

Acknowledgments

My first debt, for whatever wisdom has found its way into these pages, is to my patients, past and present. By honoring me with their trust, their unique and complex humanness, and their own wisdom, they made possible the sacred, shared learning and healing process of our work. The nature of this book also moves me to thank the teachers who most inspired and shaped the early development of my clinical, psychoanalytic self: Stephen Golding, Mark Trewartha, James Gustafson, Kenneth Newman, Merton Gill, John Gedo, Robert Galatzer-Levy, Paul Tolpin, and Marian Tolpin. Each in his or her way embodied the values that lie at the core of this book: discerning the unique and deepest therapeutic needs and strivings of our patients, and seeking to respond in human ways, which use but transcend analytic theories, including their own.

The writing of this book, including three chapters that were written before the book was conceived, has spanned a decade. Acknowledgments for Chapters 6 and 7 appear in the original journal articles. A longer draft of "Analytic Peace" (Chapter 8) served as the anchor for a 2013 IARPP (International Association of Relational Psychoanalysis and Psychotherapy) webinar, organized by Ilene Philipson, and moderated by Joye Weisel-Barth. They, and the 80+ participants, enriched my understanding and thinking, ultimately contributing to this final, published version.

A number of friends and colleagues have helped greatly, both with substantive feedback and moral support, as I have gone through the fitful process of writing this book. James William Anderson, Judy Teicholz, Donna Orange, and my book series editor, Donnel Stern, read all or most of it at different stages. Each, in her or his own way, expressed their belief in the project and helped make it a better book. My wife, Laura Kavesh not only gave me the potential space (and time) to write it; as a former professional journalist/now psychologist, she offered invaluable editorial feedback, helping me keep my writing grounded and oriented to actual human readers. Others who helped significantly with one or more individual chapters include Carla Leone, Lewis Aron, Estelle Shane, Spyros Orfanos, John Kerr, Peter Wilk, and the members of my psychoanalytic reading group in Portland, ME.

The cover art is an enhanced-image photograph by Edward A. Mason (1919–2007), my first professional mentor and life-long friend. We met fortuitously at Camp Wediko (Wediko Children's Services) in the summer of 1968, where I was a counselor and Ed was a child psychiatrist and documentary film-maker invited for the summer to make a series of educational films documenting the transformative work done mostly by college students in this remarkable therapeutic milieu. I also want to thank Ed's wife, Jean Mason, for her enthusiastic permission to use Ed's photograph for my book; and his daughter, Andrea Nolin, for her invaluable help choosing the image and modeling a preliminary design for its use on the cover.

A section of Chapter 3 is based on a section from "Identification, Repetition, and Psychological Growth: An Expansion of Relational Theory," *Psychoanalytic Psychology*, *19*: 722–738, 2002. It is reprinted with permission of the American Psychological Association.

Chapter 6 is based on "The Dialectic of Empathy and Freedom," *International Journal of Psychoanalytic Self Psychology*, *4*: 132–164, 2009. It is reprinted with permission of Taylor & Francis, LLC.

Chapter 7 is based on "The Conundrum of Self Care," *Contemporary Psychoanalysis*, *43*: 605–620, 2007. It is reprinted with permission of Taylor & Franc02is, LLC.

Introduction

An orienting principle for relational psychoanalysis[1]

When I started analytic training in the early 1990s I had been a practicing psychodynamically oriented therapist for a decade already. Sometime during my first year of training I came to two contradictory resolutions. I decided, in the service of trying to make the shift from being a psychotherapist to (my idea of) a psychoanalyst, that it would be helpful, at least for awhile, to discipline myself to saying very little, or at least much less than had been my style, to all of my patients, not just my control cases. I happened to have in my practice at the time a bright young woman, then in grad school to become a psychologist, who was naturally garrulous, quick-thinking, precociously perceptive and outspoken, and generally very engaging. Despite the temptation to join her in her quick-witted pace, I must have basically stuck to my inner pledge and done more listening than talking. Years later, when reflecting about the course of our by-then proven and highly productive therapy, she said that my relative silence and anonymity in the first few years was exactly what she had needed, given that her father had been so toxically intrusive and controlling.

The other, more or less opposite resolution I made to myself during that first year of training was that, no matter what the technical dictates putatively involved in becoming and being a "real" psychoanalyst, I would continue to trust my therapeutic instincts and personal style, and do whatever felt right, and whatever I sensed a patient needed.[2] This resolution proved helpful with my second control case—another young woman in training to be a therapist, whose relational instincts and judgment, both in her personal and professional life, seemed to me to be almost always on target, but who, given her history, was too insecure to trust her own good judgment. Consequently, a transference developed wherein she demanded constant reassurance from me in the form of saying what I really thought about her inclinations, decisions, and actions. If I hedged at all, or gave her anything like the usual analytic dodge, her anxiety rapidly escalated, as did her insistence that I tell her what I really thought before she left that day! She knew she was pressuring me to give her something that went against psychoanalytic dogma in that era (I was at a mainstream institute of the American Psychoanalytic Association), and she could even empathize. Sometimes, we joked about it. But when it came down to it, she was desperate and ruthless. So, despite the critical scrutiny I knew my work with her would be subjected to by the powers that be (except, thankfully, my supervisor, a self psychologist who was unintimidated by analytic authority and encouraged me to do what I felt she needed), I mostly did as she asked and gave her my opinions straight up, which were almost always authentically affirming of her own instincts. Whenever I did, which was at least once in every session, her anxiety immediately dissipated and she felt emboldened to go out and think or do whatever felt right to her. Over the two years I had with her, her confidence and sense of personal agency grew enormously, such that, by the time she left the state for a romance that seemed very promising, she expressed confidence that she was doing the right thing, no longer needing my validation. Subsequent correspondence confirmed her continuing and growing happiness and sense of fulfillment, personally and professionally. There was little doubt that, the psychoanalytic "rules" notwithstanding, my constant reassurance had been a primary change agent in this analytic case.

Of course both of these clinical stories are over-simplifications. There was much more going on in both treatments than can be captured by a single principle; indeed, the dense complexity of analytic interaction is one of the major themes of this book.[3] But the core truth they are intended to dramatize is the deceptively simple one that our main job as psychoanalysts and dynamic psychotherapists is to give our patients the specific kinds of help they need to move toward and achieve their therapeutic and developmental aims, both explicit and implicit, as they emerge, evolve, and become articulated within the analytic relationship. (See also Bacal, 1998, 2011.) In a sense, the universe of psychoanalytic theories and theories of technique constitute a very large and complex users' manual, the purpose of which is to offer understandings of the mind, and clinical approaches based on those understandings, all in the service of a single objective: to be able to give our patients the kinds of therapeutic experience they need in order to achieve the personal aims for which they have come to us seeking analytic help. (See also Renik, 2006.) Unfortunately, this pragmatic reason for our existence as a profession can get obscured by our love for and attachments to our theories. In a seminar I attended in the 1970s with Carl Whitaker, the famed and brilliantly outrageous family therapist, he was caricaturing the various mental health professions. "Psychoanalysts," he quipped, "mistake theory for mother's milk!"

Confusing the means with the end and mistaking the part for the whole

My version would be that psychoanalysts are prone to *confusing the means with the end*: That is, the goal of offering patients the unique forms of help they need to achieve their own therapeutic objectives can subtly shift to helping them attain an ideal end state envisioned by the analyst's theory. This is a complicated issue because patients at the outset of treatment don't typically understand the nature of the underlying psychodynamics that are responsible for the symptoms and problems that bring them to seek therapeutic help. Moreover, not only the patient but the analyst as well can get caught up in working to rid the patient of her[4] symptoms, leading into frustrating therapeutic *cul-de-sacs* (Ogden & Gabbard, 2010). Our theories address these underlying dynamics and impasses, empowering analysts with understandings, ways of being and apprehending, and techniques that can help transform them. But, as useful as the theories are, if analysts adopt them as templates imposed upon the analytic process such that the *telos* of therapy becomes the alteration of the underlying dynamics as prescribed by the theory rather than the co-creation of a process uniquely fitted to each patient's therapeutic aims and needs, the analysis will have subtly reduced the patient to a category, and lost touch with her radical uniqueness—her "face," as the ethical philosopher, Emmanuel Levinas (1969), characterized the unique individuality of every human sufferer. (See also Orange, 2011).

The themes in this book are intended to serve as a corrective to this pervasive tendency—a tendency I have been susceptible to myself, given my own love of analytic theories in general, and certain ones in particular. The corrective comes from trying to reorient the reader's attention to the construct of *needed relationships*—our efforts to discern and provide the specific kinds of analytic help each of our patients needs, both in the present analytic moment and cumulatively over time. Although an analyst's capacity to do this is grounded in knowledge of psychoanalytic theories, the theories themselves are only imperfect tools and maps to be employed in the service of the patient, and our use of them should be driven and shaped by emergent processes unique to each patient, dyad, and analytic field (Baranger & Baranger, 1961–1962/2009).

A related problem to confusing the means with the end is that of *mistaking the part for the whole.* This refers to the tendency among analytic theorists and their followers to enshrine a particular principle or set of principles of therapeutic action implied by a given theory as the foundational and universal path to psychoanalytic transformation. Many analytic clinicians, especially those strongly identified with a particular theorist or school, are not only comfortable with, but see distinct advantages in, working predominantly within a single theory or small group of theories. I have come to believe that this philosophy is increasingly untenable given the now enormous and rapidly expanding universe of psychoanalytic theories, ideas, and frames of reference, and the increasingly complex interactions among them (S. Stern, 2009b; Chapter 2 in this book).

In an earlier psychoanalytic era this error was more understandable since there were as yet only a few theories to choose from. But when contemporary authors continue to position their theoretical and therapeutic ideas as though they constitute the essence of psychoanalysis, it has at least three problematic consequences related to three inter-related meanings of "mistaking the part for the whole": (1) The theorist is not taking into account the total universe of psychoanalytic thought, which contains many compelling and competing ideas "not dreamed of in their philosophy"; (2) The author's theory and associated techniques at best only address certain aspects of our patients' psyches and problems—only one part of the elephant—never the infinitely complex whole; and (3) positioning a certain technical principle or approach as universally optimal inclines us to think about the analyst's participation in terms of categories or types of participation rather than as a more holistic relational response to the patient in all of her unique, multi-dimensional, constantly evolving, nonlinear complexity.

Some of the more familiar categories of participation are: The analyst *interprets* (Freud); the analyst engages in *empathic-introspective inquiry* (Kohut, Stolorow); the analyst *holds* (Winnicott, Slochower); the analyst *contains* (Bion); the analyst *discloses* (e.g., Ferenczi, Bollas, Davies, Renik); the analyst *is authentic or personally expressive* (e.g., Mitchell, Ehrenberg, Hoffman); the analyst *recognizes* (Benjamin); the analyst *negotiates* (Pizer); the analyst engages in *reverie* or *waking dreaming* (Bion, Ogden); the analyst communicates at the level of *implicit relational knowing* (Lyons-Ruth, Boston Change Process Study Group); the analyst seeks to foster *connectedness* (Geist); the analyst engages in *self-state sharing* (Bromberg). These categories of therapist participation and the theories which underpin them are indispensible. Each one offers a different "vertex" (Bion, 1962) (read: frame of reference) from which to organize clinical data, and each has its own associated implications for the kinds of participation our patients most need. But because we have learned to think in terms of these categories, *we don't tend to think of the analytic relationship more holistically*, which seems ironic for analysts and therapists who define their theoretical orientation as *relational*.

Having received analytic training during a period (the 1990s) when my institute, like most others, had begun to adopt a comparative psychoanalytic pedagogic approach, my philosophy has always tended toward theoretical heterogeneity and synthesis. Influenced by the contextualist epistemology of our era, I think of all psychoanalytic theories as products of their particular authors' personal subjectivities and histories (Stolorow & Atwood, 1979; Anderson, 2005), and the particular historical/cultural contexts within which their ideas emerged. Because of the unique genius of our major theorists, their core insights contributed something unique, essential, and timeless (or at least possessing a very long shelf life) to our overall understanding of the human psyche and analytic process. At the same time, these insights, in order to remain fully relevant and alive, have had to be continually re-evaluated, re-contextualized and reinvented by subsequent theorists, usually within more complex theoretical frameworks, and always in idiomatic ways that are the products of *those* theorists' personalities and historical/cultural contexts. Because of the more or less infinite complexity of the human psyche, I think all of our theorists, even the geniuses, have only been privileged to see some part of that complexity—never the whole—a part that became "visible" in their particular historical context.[5] Thus, my inclination is to find value, but also limitations, in any of our theorists' insights, and to try to fit the insights I value (like pieces in a mysterious, four dimensional, ever-morphing puzzle) into my own evolving and increasingly complex understanding and vision of the whole.

A complex illustration: Stephen Mitchell's relational-conflict theory of therapeutic action

In Mitchell's 1997 book, *Influence and Autonomy in Psychoanalysis*, the second chapter was tellingly entitled, "*The* Therapeutic Action: A New Look" (emphasis added). In it Mitchell begins by arguing that each of the major psychoanalytic theories has had its own idea of the "royal road" to effecting analytic transformation. For example, in the Freudian model it is *interpretation*, whereas in the Kohutian model it is *empathic immersion and understanding.* He offers persuasive clinical examples in which the patient simply absorbs these forms of analyst participation into her rigid, pre-existing patterns of experiencing and relating—patterns that are refractory to the analyst's efforts to do more of the same (i.e., more interpreting or attempting to make empathically attuned statements), even after incorporating the new information gleaned from the patient's original response. Mitchell argues that the problem with these earlier models was that they assumed, when it came to therapeutic action, that one size could fit all, whereas in fact patients can always unconsciously find ways to incorporate any of the analyst's therapeutic efforts into pre-existing experiential categories and thus draw the analyst into what is essentially a repetition or variation of the relational difficulties for which she is seeking help.

Mitchell's argument up to this point is, in my view, brilliant, and has remained with me as a lesson in the limitations inherent in *any* single theory or technical model, including ones I am fond of. However, he then goes on to assert that the relational model he has developed and is advocating solves the problem of the earlier models because it is non-prescriptive and grounded in the unique dynamics of each patient and dyad. According to his argument, every patient can be counted on to enlist the analyst in some form of unconscious repetitive enactment; in fact, Mitchell believed this needed to occur for a treatment to be fully engaged. Therefore, he argued, therapeutic action and progress could only come from the analyst struggling to find unique, emergent ways to engage and confront enactments "from within" the transference-countertransference field; to find a unique and authentic "voice" with which to speak to the analysand, which the analysand could experience as "something new"—i.e., as a liberation from the constraints of her "old object" patterns of relational engagement. Mitchell argued that the advantage of this approach was that it did not fall prey to the limitations of the single-principle theories of therapeutic action in the older models because the solution in each case—the "new object" experience that lay at the core of therapeutic action and transformation—had to be uniquely found with each patient, and found from within the inevitable, co-created re-enactments.

These were seminal insights that laid the foundation of a new theory of analytic interaction and cure, and a new paradigm of analytic thought. Yet, despite Mitchell's attempt to escape and transcend this very problem, his model also falls prey to the limitations of a theory grounded in a single principle, although in a somewhat different sense. In my experience at least, while the kind of relational sequence he describes—from repetition or enactment to liberation and new experience—may be the crux of some treatments, it is by no means central in the analytic process of all treatments. For example, I would not say that Mitchell's model of therapeutic action was centrally involved in either of the treatments I referenced at the beginning of this chapter. It was not my experience that the needed forms of interaction that evolved in these cases emerged from earlier repetitive enactments. I think such repetitions could easily have occurred had I been more active and knowing with the first patient, or had I stuck to the analytic rules and frustrated my second patient's need for reassurance. It was undoubtedly true that there were elements of repetition or enactment in both cases, even as the dominant experience was one of positive, needed engagement, and even that these repetitive elements contributed in some necessary way to each patient's therapeutic engagement (Hoffman, 1998). Were I conducting those treatments today I would be trying to observe the interaction with an eye to this possibility, always wondering if there might be something important "going on around here" (Levenson, 1983) that I was missing. But I would have been in trouble with these patients had I been focusing in a major way on trying to detect enactments I was certain *must* be going on, rather than trusting my sense of who they were, what they needed from me, and what was happening in the interaction. I would say that the success of these treatments does support part of Mitchell's theory—a part with which I agree: namely, that both patients experienced me as providing a *new relational experience uniquely fitted to their therapeutic needs and which contrasted in critical ways with the traumatizing, toxic experiences of their childhoods*. But significantly, I didn't arrive at either mode of relating through any particular theory that I was aware of using. This was obviously true in the first case. But even in the second case, which generally I was trying to conduct along self-psychological lines, the critical mode of interaction—a mode which, in my now 30-plus years of doing psychotherapy, was unlike any other in which I have ever engaged—emerged from the unique needs and exigencies of the patient in the context of our particular analytic system and process.

My purpose in using Mitchell's theory as an example is not to single him out for criticism; indeed, as I have already suggested, he is in good company. Rather it is to illustrate the subtle ways that even seminal theories can mistake the part for the whole. This pitfall actually seems to be endemic to psychoanalytic theorizing. The major psychoanalytic theorists, beginning with Freud, have aimed to generate understandings that are better fitted to the problems and therapeutic needs of psychoanalytic patients than previous understandings. Even when the theories ostensibly grew out of attempts to better understand specific categories of patients, most seem to expand in scope until, ultimately, they are seen by their authors, or the authors' followers, to be encompassing, foundational theories, generalizable to all analytic patients. Winnicott and Kohut both initially developed their respective theories of the self to expand the scope of psychoanalytic understanding beyond the Oedipal neuroses to more serious (pre-Oedipal) character pathology. And Bion's theory of thinking and dreaming grew, in part, out of his experience with psychotics—i.e., patients with disorders of thought and an inability to dream. Psychoanalysis has benefitted from this expansionist tendency. These theorists really were onto something much larger than their original projects. Believing in the truth of their insights, they aimed to place psychoanalysis in general on a sounder, more reality-based, more clinically effective footing. I believe they accomplished this and in so doing opened up whole new dimensions of psychological and therapeutic understanding—understandings that probably *are* applicable to *many* psychoanalytic patients. In this sense the impulse to discover or work toward a grand, overarching psychoanalytic theory has mostly benefitted our patients and the field as a whole.

But ironically, this very evolution and proliferation of compelling but diverse theories and understandings, in combination with the post-modern, critical-contextualist sensibility and its suspiciousness of essences of any kind, has led to our current, humbling appreciation of the complexity of the human psyche-in-context and the analytic process, as well as the inherent contextual limitations of any given theory. It has also led us into a collective conceptual, epistemological space in which our theories themselves have become more self-reflexive such that they *theorize* the necessity of being aware of one's relationship to and use of theory, given the inherent limitations, and potential misuse, of any theory. Thus Stolorow and his collaborators (e.g., Stolorow & Atwood, 1992; Brandchaft, 2010) have sensitized us to the fact that our theories are, in effect, part of countertransference (part of the analyst's subjective organizing principles) and can interfere with (even as they make possible) empathic connection with our patients. In a similar vein, Orange (e.g., 2011) has repeatedly urged us to "hold our theories lightly."

An orienting principle and mantra

In this book the phrase, *needed relationship*, is an umbrella term and orienting principle for the ideas I have begun to develop in the previous sections. As an orienting principle it prompts relational-analytic clinicians to always be holding loosely in mind the question, "What does the patient need from me?" as an implicit mantra—a "North Star"—for navigating the fast-moving, often murky and turbulent, currents of the analytic process. Although the question is simple, the answers are always complex, often elusive, and rarely certain. Both the principle and the mantra contain deeply embedded paradoxes and dialectical tensions, which I try to open up in different ways throughout this book. One such paradox concerns the analytic therapist's relationship to theory. On one hand, the question, "What does the patient need from me?" can only be answered, in an analytic context, through each therapist's particular internalization and integration of analytic (and related) theories. On the other hand, the question underlines the primacy of each patient's unique therapeutic needs as co-constructed within each analytic dyad. Thus, the needed relationship, in the present analytic moment and over time, always transcends theory while potentially, implicitly, drawing upon multiple theories as "selected" by the needs of the moment. (See Bacal, 2011, for a similar viewpoint regarding the selective use and adaptation of multiple theories to fit the unique needs of each patient and dyad.)

This paradox makes explicit the daunting complexity of the contemporary relational analyst's job. One way to capture this complexity is to imagine the analytic therapist-at-work as serving a bridging function between two enormously complex dynamic systems: that of the patient-analyst dyad as constituted within its analytic field (Coburn, 2014; Baranger & Baranger, 1961–1962/2009); and that of the rapidly expanding and increasingly complex universe of psychoanalytic theories and ideas, as selected, experienced, processed, and reinvented by each analytic therapist. The art of psychoanalysis in our psychoanalytic era may be synonymous with performing this bridging function well-enough, where "well-enough" also implies the final step of translating all of this complexity into authentic, "simply human" responses to our patients' human needs of the moment, and communicating those responses in language (verbal and implicit) that is progressively fitted to what the patient is able to hear and use. In this book, guided by the deceptively simple concept of needed relationship, I try to make explicit my approach to thinking about and trying to perform these functions with my patients.

A core premise of this approach, which one might think would be axiomatic in relational psychoanalysis, is that it is the analytic relationship, *as a whole*, which is curative. Relational psychoanalytic theory has illuminated many dimensions of the analytic process and therapeutic action. But surprisingly, the analytic relationship itself—its full complexity—as experienced in the present moment and cumulatively over time, is rarely theorized. Of course, I don't purport to grasp the total complexity of analytic relationships. Such complexity is infinite and, at best, can only be represented by abstractions such as Bion's (1967, 1970) concept of "O." My aim is considerably more modest: to identify principles that orient clinicians to the analytic patient, dyad, and process in *holistic* ways, even as we are simultaneously cognizant of particular dimensions of experience as highlighted in our various analytic theories and models of the mind.

The concept of relational *fittedness*, first introduced by the infancy researcher and theorist, Louis Sander (1995, 2002, 2008), is a central organizing principle of this book. I, like Sander, view progressive fittedness as a developing property of productive patient/analyst dyadic systems analogous to the achievement of progressive fittedness between a caregiver and baby (or really child of any age) in the service of helping the child master developmental tasks. Achieving fittedness, as Sander imagined it, "can be thought of as a way of representing how one individual comes to *savor the wholeness of another* . . . the critical condition for the reorganization of both interacting partners as they progress toward new integration" (2008, p. 169; emphasis added). Sander (2008) draws the analogy between the mother-infant and therapist-patient systems in his papers, but does not flesh out its full implications for clinical practice. A central aim of this book is to pick up where Sander left off and develop further the complex clinical implications of this paradigm.[6]

One implication of adopting a fittedness perspective is that the things we actually say and do with patients often do not fall neatly into established categories of analyst participation. Rather, they are *contoured* to the patient and the analytic moment, guided by one's implicit effort to *meet* the patient at the point of analytic urgency, taking into account the current state of the patient, the therapist, and their system. The clinical examples offered throughout this book are intended to demonstrate this approach and sensibility. Different from many psychoanalytic texts presenting theories of technique, this book offers no clear take-away method or way of thinking to provide guidance with challenging cases. What you will find instead is me drawing on multiple psychoanalytic theories and modes of participation in unpredictable, idiomatic, spontaneous ways, as I attempt to fit my interventions to the current, usually complex, analytic situation. I hope these diverse clinical examples have the effect of helping readers feel freer to find your own creative voices and idioms of participation as you seek to respond to the unique needs of each patient, in each session and analytic moment.

Nine principles of needed analytic relationships

The following nine principles constitute the scaffolding of an orientation to the analytic process viewed as the progressive co-creation of needed relationships:

1 Every analytic patient and dyad is *unique*; thus the needed relationship(s) that emerge in each treatment are also unique.
2 The *telos* of analytic treatment is *progressive fittedness* (Sander, 1995, 2008) between the patient's evolving therapeutic needs and the relationship that emerges to meet those needs.
3 Progressive fittedness involves progressive *understanding*, progressive shaping of the ways we learn to *listen, process, and speak* with each patient, and progressive fittedness in the *forms and qualities of relational engagement* that emerge in each treatment. Understanding ("truth") and relational engagement are viewed as inseparable and as operating synergistically.

4 Achieving progressive fittedness does not necessarily mean meeting the patient's needs on the terms that the patient is stating them or complying with some fantasized response that the patient is enactively "pulling for." Rather, it means *co-creating the therapeutic conditions* that best enable the patient to work and move toward her mostly implicit therapeutic/developmental aims as these become actualized and articulated within the analytic setting over time.
5 Achieving fittedness in each treatment requires considerable *improvisational freedom* on the part of analytic therapists, balanced, of course, with the discipline necessary for establishing and holding an analytic frame and shepherding an analytic process. Fittedness, whatever forms it might take in a given moment, session, or period of treatment, is thus an *emergent* phenomenon within a fluid, evolving, non-linear dynamic system.
6 At the same time, there may be an intersubjective *tendency toward progressive fittedness*—a property of patient/analyst systems that are functioning well enough—just as there may be such a tendency in good-enough caregiver/infant systems (Sander, 2008). Such a system-tendency implies *unconscious* as well as conscious intention, which I think of as the *forward edge* (Tolpin, 2002) *of the relational unconscious.*
7 Therapeutic interventions in the service of achieving progressive fittedness are primarily *patient-driven (or perhaps, dyad-driven) rather than theory-driven*. That is to say, the concepts of needed relationship and progressive fittedness are intended to be relatively *theoretically neutral or empty*.
8 At the same time, we do, of course, rely on our theories to understand our patients, including our understanding of what they need from us. It's just that no single theory can, in our psychoanalytic era, be regarded as foundational or sufficient. The universe of theories and psychoanalytic frames of reference has become enormously and increasingly complex, with extremely complex interactions among them; *thus our relationship to this constantly evolving, swirling universe in the context of our interactions with our patients can usefully be regarded as a complex, non-linear dynamic system in its own right.*
9 The psychoanalytic relationship (within its analytic field) is a complex *transformational medium*—a kind of relational Petri dish in a constant state of flux—with many elements in fluid interaction. This metaphor, which seeks to capture the dense complexity of the analytic process,

stands in contrast to theory-based characterizations emphasizing single principles (or even multiple principles) as the essential mutative factor(s). The elements are always changing and evolving, and there are always new elements emerging as part of the co-creative, improvisational project of achieving progressive fittedness in the service of facilitating the patient's desired transformation and growth.

Like-minded ideas

Although no other analytic author formulates these principles in exactly the same way I do, numerous others throughout the history of the field have articulated similar ideas. The following represents a sampling, which, taken as a group, adds force to the meta-theoretical position I am advocating. That is, I believe this current of thought has been present in psychoanalysis since its inception.

Freud (1912b), in his "Recommendations to Physicians on the Technique of Psycho-analysis," famously wrote:

> I think I am well-advised . . . to call these rules "recommendations" and not to claim any unconditional acceptance for them. The extraordinary diversity of the psychical constellations concerned, the plasticity of all mental processes and the wealth of determining factors oppose any mechanization of the technique . . .
>
> (p. 123)

Ferenczi (1928), in his essay "The Elasticity of Psycho-analytic Technique," echoed Freud's sentiment but with an early "relational" addition:

> A patient of mine once spoke of the "elasticity of analytic technique," a phrase which I fully accept. The analyst, like an elastic band, must yield to the patient's pull, but without ceasing to pull in his own direction, so long as one position or the other has not been conclusively demonstrated to be untenable.
>
> (p. 95)

Jumping forward in time to our contemporary era, the beginning of which I date to Winnicott and Bion, I view the following ideas, many of which I will return to in later chapters, as offered in a similar vein:

Winnicott's (1965) concept of "adaptation to need," which, in an analytic context, means adaptation of the analyst's technique to the patient's unique therapeutic needs.

Bion's (1967, 1970) paradoxical injunction to approach every analytic session "without memory or desire"—that is, without preconception or the need to make something happen—so as to be maximally receptive to the unique psychic realities of every patient and session; and his related (1987) advice to approach every session with a patient as if it were the first session.

Ogden's (2009) statement (influenced by these precepts from Bion) that it is the analyst's "role to create psychoanalysis freshly with each patient in each session of the analysis."

Kohut's (1984) introduction of the concepts of "experience-near" theory and "empathic immersion," both intended to bring the analyst closer to apprehending the patient's unique subjective experince in each analytic moment and hour.

Bacal's concepts of "optimal responsiveness" (1998) and therapeutic "specificity" (Bacal, 2011), which are especially close to the principles and perspective I am developing in this book.

Sander's (1995, 2008) concepts of "specificity of recognition," "specificity of connection," and "fittedness."

D.B. Stern's (2003) admonition, following Gadamer (1965), to strive for awareness of our "prejudices" in our attempt to take into account the unique individuality of every patient (her "otherness") within the context of the unfolding dialogue.

Orange's (1995, 2011) recommendation (also informed by Gadamer, as well as by Levinas, 1969), that analysts "hold their theories lightly" in the service of apprehending, and allowing themselves to be "compelled" by, the unique nature of each patient's struggles and needs.

Bass' (2007) more elastic re-envisioning of the analytic frame as "containing, reflecting, and blending aspects of the two separate and unique subjectivities engaged in an analytic process" (p. 13).

The principle of "autocatalysm" from psychoanalytic applications of non-linear dynamic systems theory, according to which "the agent

> of change emerges as a product and property of the relational system itself" (Coburn, 2014, Kindle Edition, Introduction: "Attitudes," Attitude 4).

I view this group of concepts and statements as sharing, explicitly or implicitly, the superordinate principle that every patient, dyad, and analytic process is unique; hence the nature of every analytic needed relationship is also unique, and, I would add, uniquely complex. It is also true that many of these analytic thinkers have developed more specific models of the mind and principles of therapeutic action. There is no contradiction here so long as the authors in question, or at least *we*, are not holding up their specific ideas about therapeutic action as the universal and foundational royal road to psychoanalytic cure. We need our models of the mind and therapeutic action in order to do psychoanalysis, but we need to use them without confusing the means with the end or mistaking the part for the whole.

Plan of the book

In Chapter 1 I propose the concept of needed relationship as an organizing framework for relational psychoanalysis, articulating what I believe to be the advantages of thinking about the analytic process in this way. I also introduce Sander's (1995, 2002, 2008) principles of "specificity of recognition," "specificity of connection," "moments of meeting," and "progressive fittedness," and the philosophy that underlies them, as highly resonant with my ideas about needed relationships. I then begin the process, fleshed out in subsequent chapters, of imagining how his concepts, which grew out of his longitudinal studies of mother-infant interaction, can be adapted to the context of adult psychoanalytic therapy relationships. I argue that the full implementation of his principles in adult psychotherapy can only occur through the intermediate area (Winnicott, 1971a) of psychoanalytic theories. It is our theories that instruct us in how to meet our patients in spaces where being met is an alien, distrusted experience, which patients may misread, avoid, negate, or attack even as they unconsciously long for and seek it.

In Chapter 2, I take a step back and look at our evolving relationship to psychoanalytic theory, given the increasing complexity of the nature of our theories and the interactions among them. I argue that the terms have changed even since a few decades ago. Whereas then we could still meaningfully speak of theoretical plurality and comparative psychoanalysis, now, with the proliferation of theories, part-theories, and innovative frames of reference, and the ways these innovations alter and render more complex our relationship to all theories, past and present, it seems more realistic to think of our relationship to the theoretical universe as a non-linear dynamic, increasingly complex, system. Yet this increasing complexity, paradoxically, brings us closer and closer to the "live pulse" of the clinical exchange and makes possible progressively fitted, "simply human" responses to our patients.

Chapters 3 and 4 examine the vicissitudes of the concept of progressive fittedness in the adult analytic situation. To realize the clinical potential of the concept in its full depth requires understanding certain core paradoxes and dialectics that are implicit to its application. Having explored these in Chapter 3, in Chapter 4 I examine the intriguing possibility that there is a natural *tendency toward progressive fittedness* in adult analytic dyads comparable to that which can be observed in well-enough functioning mother-infant pairs. Such a tendency implies that there is a forward-edge tendency (Tolpin, 2002) not only intrinsic to the patient's individual unconscious but to the relational unconscious as well.

Chapter 5, long enough to be a monograph in its own right, is an in-depth examination of the relationship between *understanding* and *relational engagement* in the analytic process. The chapter begins with a highly condensed and selective overview of relational thinking on this topic, focusing on the question of where each author or school comes down on the question of the how these two dimensions of analytic interaction (understanding and engagement) are conceptualized, prioritized, and integrated in their models.

The chapter then turns to a specific consideration of the trend in contemporary relational thinking emphasizing the centrality of interaction in the register of "implicit relational knowing." I argue, from a number of different vantage points, that, while the recognition of the pervasiveness and importance of implicit communication in the analytic relationship has been a major contribution, the bifurcation of analytic interaction into implicit/non-verbal/unsymbolized/right-brain-to-right-brain *versus* explicit/cognitive/verbal-symbolic/left-brain-to-left-brain interaction, and the implication that the former is primary and more central to therapeutic action than the latter, are misguided and illogical inferences which miss the larger trend toward recognizing the essential synergy between these two inseparable modes of experiencing and engaging. In the final section of the chapter I outline my own current synthesis and offer a brief, ordinary clinical example as illustration.

Chapters 6 and 7 each take up particular kinds of dialectical tension pertinent to the co-creation of needed relationships with our patients. In Chapter 6 I apply dialectical thinking to the Kohutian concept of empathy. I argue that self-psychologists' commitment to the principle of empathic inquiry and attunement represents a particular analytic *intention*, or, in Bion's (1970) language, a *desire*. As such, from a Bionian perspective, it has the same problem as any therapeutic desire—namely, that it limits the analyst's *freedom* to apprehend and experience the analytic encounter without preconception or any particular therapeutic intention or need. Grounding my thinking in both Bion's and Winnicott's ideas, I propose that analytic empathy needs to be held in dialectical tension with the principle of analytic freedom, which I define.

In Chapter 7 I focus on a particular kind of clinical problem—the needs of patients who present with serious (worrisome) problems in their self-care. With such patients the analytically needed relationship often must go beyond empathy and interpretation to include confronting, directive and instructive forms of intervention, which I refer to as "concerned action". I posit a dialectical tension between *empathic recognition* and *concerned action* implicitly held by parents in relation to their children's' development, and suggested for analytic therapists working with patients with self-care issues. Usually, patients presenting with such difficulties have experienced a breakdown in this necessary dialectical tension in their families of origin, and thus need it to be re-established in treatment. I begin Chapter 7 by contextualizing these ideas meta-theoretically as one version of a more general phenomenon: that there are really two kinds of need embedded in many of our patients' struggles: *subjectively felt* and *objectively perceived* needs.

The book concludes, in Chapter 8, with an extended meditation on my concept of *analytic peace*.

Notes

1 The terms psychoanalysis or analysis, psychoanalyst or analyst, and analytic relationship, as used throughout this book, are intended to be inclusive of all analytic psychotherapies, and analytically oriented psychotherapists. The term

"relational psychoanalysis" (with a small "r") is meant to be inclusive of all relational theories, as opposed to Relational (with a capital "R"), which will be used to refer to the so-called New York Relational school.

2 These two apparently contradictory resolutions could be seen as an early variation of Hoffman's (1998) dialectic of "analytic ritual and discipline vs. spontaneity and personal expressiveness."

3 It could have been the case, for example, that what was transformative in my direct reassurances (and occasional questions, challenges, and disagreements) with the second patient was not the content of my feedback per se but something more complex in our total communication, including: (1) the implicit dimension of how I experienced and processed not only the patient's questions but the patient herself as she asked each question; and (2) how I formed my responses to the questions (both the words and the "music") to fit my sense of what was needed in the moment. And it was likely the case with the first patient that my relatively quiet presence was not simply "neutral" but rather what Grossmark (2012b) has described as a form of "unobtrusively" attuned participation: " . . . a tactful and connected 'silence,' a 'with-ness' (Reis, 2011, cited in Grossmark 2012b) that does not intrude on the patient's ownership of their sensations and their own particular experience of the analyst, by knowing more than the patient or even offering the patient more than they create themselves in the moment." (p. 633)

4 Singular male and female pronouns are used interchangeably throughout this book to represent indeterminate antecedents.

5 In a personal communication (2016), my psychobiographer friend Jim Anderson alerted me to the fact that William James had made the following, strikingly similar statement in 1908: "[N]either the whole of good nor the whole of truth is revealed to any singular observer, although each observer gains a partial superiority from the particular position in which he stands." Drawing on James and others, Jim takes a similar position in his own paper (Anderson, 2005).

6 Many of Sander's ideas have informed the Boston Change Process Study Group's evolving understanding of the analytic process (e.g., D.N. Stern et al., 1998; BCPSG 2008, 2010, 2013). While there are significant areas of agreement between their model and mine, I also take these ideas in some different (and in certain ways opposing) directions.

Chapter 1

Needed relationships and psychoanalytic healing

The phrase *needed relationship*, in its broadest meaning, refers to the fact that the psychoanalytic relationship is first and foremost a special human relationship that forms over time between patient and analyst: It is this special relationship that carries the healing power of psychoanalytic treatment and makes psychoanalysis unique among the healing vocations. Whereas in professions such as medicine and spiritual teaching, and in non-relational psychotherapies, the relationship between the persons giving and receiving treatment or guidance is usually seen as an important *vehicle* for delivering needed help, in psychoanalysis the analytic relationship itself *is* the primary treatment agent (see also Mitchell, 1997). This is, and always has been, true despite the fact that Freud, and decades of classically minded analysts who followed his lead, wanted to view the relationship between patient and analyst as essentially similar to that between a medical doctor and patient. The treatment relied on the patient *experiencing* the analyst *as if* the two parties had a real and important relationship "in the transference," and it was recognized that the analyst was vulnerable to reactively falling in with that illusion or fantasy "in the countertransference." But the analyst needed to remain clear that the patient's experience was indeed an illusion grounded in "pathogenic instincts" (Freud, 1914, p. 154)—an illusion which, in order to be used therapeutically, could not be shared or indulged.[1] Nonetheless, despite his cautions and disavowals, time and subsequent theoretical advances have made clear that one of Freud's two most significant acts of genius (the other being his discovery of the unconscious), was his creation of a human relationship with new and unique therapeutic properties.

It was not until the mid-twentieth century and the advent of an increasingly explicit relational psychoanalytic paradigm in the writings of

Fairbairn, Winnicott, Balint, Sullivan, Bion, Kohut, Loewald, and others (Greenberg & Mitchell, 1983) that the true nature and healing potential of Freud's invention began to be more fully understood and actualized. Since then, especially with the intersubjective or relational turn in American psychoanalytic theory that began in the early 1980s, there has been an increasing focus on the therapeutic potential of analysis as a multidimensional human relationship, and with this focus an elaboration of the many ways that this unique relationship can respond to the therapeutic needs of a wider and wider scope (A. Freud, 1954; Stone, 1954) of patients with increasingly diverse forms of psychopathology, or, as I prefer to think of them, forms of personal struggle. In this book my aim is to further illuminate the complex and mysterious properties of the analytic relationship as a healing agent by opening up the concept of needed relationship and exploring its implications in various contexts.

In my original, more limited use of the phrase (S. Stern, 1994), the *needed relationship* referred to the positive, "new object" dimension of the transference-countertransference relationship as opposed to the *repeated relationship*, which referred to the negative, "old object" dimension. The phrase, in that context, had echoes of Kohut's (1971, 1977, 1984) (developmentally needed) selfobject relationship, Winnicott's (1965) therapeutic principle of the analyst's adaptation (of technique) to the patient's developmental needs, and Gedo's (1979) recognition that some patients have developmental gaps in their acquisition of essential "psychological skills" and thus have a need for a uniquely analytic form of "instruction" in those skills. One of my major points in that paper was that the unconscious communications and pulls of patients in psychoanalytic treatment are not only in the direction of enacting old problematic patterns of relational engagement (e.g., Mitchell, 1988, 1997); patients also unconsciously pull for or signal (directly or indirectly) the kinds of responses they long for or need from the analyst. Accordingly, analysts, unconsciously (and/or consciously) responding to *this* kind of pressure, may find themselves engaging in more positive forms of enactment.[2]

I still believe this to be the case, and find that this understanding remains insufficiently incorporated into contemporary Relational theory, which continues to focus disproportionately on problematic enactments. Consequently, in this book I am still advocating for more of a balance in how we think about the analytic process and therapeutic action. However, in the present book the phrase needed relationship, while retaining some of its earlier meaning, has expanded to refer to *the healing aspects of the analytic relationship in all of its therapeutic complexity*.

The contemporary Relational focus on repetition (Mitchell, 1988, 1997), enactments (Levenson, 1972, 1983; Bromberg, 1998, 2011; D.B. Stern, 2010), impasses (Stolorow & Atwood, 1992), doer/done-to complementarities (Benjamin, 2004), subjugating thirds (Ogden, 1994), crunches (Russell, 2006), and other forms of difficulty caused by conflicts and disjunctions between and within the patient's and the analyst's subjectivities, has been critical to the development of powerful new understandings and clinical approaches within the Relational paradigm. At the same time, it has given Relational psychoanalysis a pathology-oriented cast—a disproportionate emphasis on what Tolpin (2002) termed "the trailing edge" as opposed to "the forward edge" of the patient's moment-to-moment states and self-presentation, and the analytic process as a whole. One might glean from the mainstream Relational literature (with many notable exceptions) that the needed analytic relationship is primarily defined as a set of strategies for recognizing, withstanding, and recovering from or transforming enactments and other forms of relational turbulence, rather than a more balanced view in which recognizing and coping with enactments is only part of a broader conception of what our patients need from us in the service of their treatment aims and psychological growth. In my experience, while working with enactments may be one of the hardest parts of analysis (thus warranting the attention they have received), it is not the biggest or, necessarily, the most important part. The concept of needed relationship is intended as a more balanced overall conceptual and therapeutic frame for relational psychoanalysis.

One of the gains from this reorientation is that it sensitizes analytic clinicians to the fact that new, needed therapeutic experiences in analysis have their own complexity and, in many analytic treatments, become more potent and resilient as they become increasingly nuanced and fitted to the unique needs of the patient. If positive or needed experiences are framed principally in terms of emergence from negative or constricting experience (conflicts, enactments and the like), this limits one's ability to recognize their co-created complexity, especially as they take on a life of their own and evolve over time.

I should say that the distinction I am making here between negative and positive relational experience is an over-simplification in the sense that all analytic interaction is complex and, by its nature, ambiguous (Baranger & Baranger, 1961–1962/2009). Not only is it true that problematic enactments are often accompanied by positive background elements, especially in established, productive analytic relationships, *the same interaction* can often be both positive and negative (see also Hoffman, 1998). For example, the power struggle described in the case illustration that concludes this chapter could be said to have simultaneous negative and positive elements.

I agree with Levenson (1972, 1983) that enactment is constant in analysis. I would even say that an analysis, from beginning to end, is essentially a long, complex "developmental enactment" (Orange, 2012) in the sense that it is primarily a *lived experience*, and that what is transformative is a function of the unique forms of lived experience that analysis potentially offers (co-creates). Where I disagree with Levenson is with the assumption that *what* is enacted is always a transform of the problems under consideration at the level of verbal inquiry, or even problems of any kind. That is simply not my experience, and I believe that examining analytic interaction through a lens that is biased in the direction of seeing the difficulty, rather than a totality that includes the remedy as well as the difficulty, runs the risk of interfering with an unfolding connectedness (Geist, 2009), thereby potentially retraumatizing the patient in ways that *are* enactive in the problematic sense.

I would argue that both the nature and the experienced quality of analytic interaction are so entangled with the ways that the analyst is holding, perceiving, interpreting, and participating in the interaction, that Levenson's (1983) extremely useful question, "What's going on around here?" (i.e., what is being enacted even as we speak), becomes a Zen-like *koan* that cannot be answered from any single frame of reference or vertex (Bion, 1962). For example, if I approach the unfolding analytic engagement with the implicit question, "What does the patient need from me?" and am experiencing, and participating in, the analytic exchange through that vertex, the nature of "what's going on here" must now include whatever effects my participating in this way have on what's going on. Similarly, if my dominant approach to the ongoing interaction is through the vertex of the question, "What's going on around here?" this also will have a particular effect on the nature of what *is* going on.

To state this issue more generally, the question I am raising is how the analyst's *intentional* orientation to the process interacts with and affects the *unintentional* dimensions of the process implied in the question, "What's going on around here?"—recognizing that the question, "What's going on around here?" *is itself* an intentional orientation to the process. My own current solution to the *koan* is that, while there are extreme, unresolvable paradoxes involved, overall the question, "What does the patient need from me?" is superordinate to the question, "What's going on around here?" but that part (though by no means all) of what the patient needs from me is to be asking the question, "What's going on here?" and employing that question to better approach the question of what the patient needs. This hierarchy tilts the analyst's primary hermeneutic from one of suspicion (Ricoeur, 1970) to one of relatively greater faith or trust (Orange, 2011) in so far as it assumes that, no matter what's going on, there is always an underlying forward-edge need (Tolpin, 2002) that is being implicitly expressed in whatever is going on.

Meta-principle and clinical reality

An admittedly elusive concept, the needed analytic relationship has meaning as both a conceptual frame or meta-principle (really, a set of principles—see Introduction) for imagining and doing analytic work, and as a descriptor of actual clinical interaction, either in the present moment of analytic exchange or cumulatively over time. At first blush, it might seem to imply a reified quality, as if one could specify a certain type of needed relationship for a given patient. While it is possible retrospectively to characterize certain patterns of interaction or processes that seem to have been most helpful to a patient over time, the analytic relationship, in fact, unfolds complexly and unpredictably, and simultaneously on different time scales: the present moment, a period of work organized around certain tensions and themes, and cumulatively over the course of treatment from beginning to end (Marks-Tarlow, 2008). Thus, as all analytic clinicians since Freud (1913) have understood, what is needed in a given moment, session, or treatment phase is complex and not specifiable in advance. The analyst is guided by her history with the patient and thus has many implicit understandings or proto-understandings (senses) of what the patient might need from her at a particular time. Moreover, the analyst is always guided implicitly by her idiomatic, evolving integration of the history of psychoanalytic ideas about needed relationships, and in this sense could probably locate her actions in a given moment within, or at least in relation to, this complex, moving, historical-conceptual frame. These senses and conceptual integrations inform what the analyst says and does but are never the whole story because the moment-to-moment, session-to-session interaction presents complex information, evokes constantly shifting meanings, and exerts constantly changing pressures, all of which call for a moment-to-moment improvisational inventiveness (Ogden, 2009).

One reason I like the concept of needed relationship is its *generality* and *relative theoretical neutrality* or *emptiness*. There is a tendency in psychoanalytic theories of therapeutic action, from at least as far back as Strachey (1934) through the present day, to take a particular therapeutic idea or set of ideas—in Strachey's case, the idea of mutative transference interpretation—and generalize it to all analytic patients and situations. As discussed in the Introduction, I think of this tendency as *mistaking the part for the whole*. The meta-theory of needed relationships invites the analyst to draw upon *all* existing theories of therapeutic action as well as unique, never-previously formulated ideas that might emerge creatively, as these might seem to apply in a given case in a given moment or period of work.

Sander's theory of progressive fittedness and specificity of recognition

To state this same idea in different language, the concept of needed relationship encourages openness, creativity, and a certain freedom (from established categories of analyst participation) in generating and attempting to fit interventions uniquely to each patient and treatment situation. (See also Bacal, 1998, 2011.) The developmental researcher and theorist, Louis Sander (e.g., 1995, 2002, 2008), proposed the concept of *fittedness* to describe the result when a good enough parent or therapist meets the child or patient in such a way that some developmental or therapeutic need or aim of the moment is met or accomplished at a new level. The achievement of fittedness involves collaboration and coordination between the two individuals (the parent or therapist doing most of the accommodating) in the service of the child's or patient's overall development: especially, in Sander's view, development of the senses of "wholeness" or "coherence," and personal agency. There is almost the implication, in Sander's account, that progressive fittedness is *an inherent property* of caregiver-and-infant as a complex system (under good enough conditions) such that the two component sub-systems (i.e., parent and infant) spontaneously move in the direction of coordination and fittedness. Listen to his frame-by-frame narrative of, and commentary on, a now often-cited video segment taken of a member of Daniel Stern's research team—a father holding his baby daughter in his arms—as he is talking informally with other members of the team, standing together on a lawn during a home visit with one of their neonatal subjects:

> . . . one sees the father glance down momentarily at the baby's face. Strangely enough, in the same frames, the infant looks up at the father's face. Then the infant's left arm, which had been hanging down over the father's left arm, begins to move upward. Miraculously in the same frame, the father's right arm, which had been hanging down at his right side, begins to move upward. Frame by frame by frame, the baby's hand and the father's hand move upward simultaneously. Finally, just as they meet over the baby's tummy, the baby's left hand grasps the little finger of the father's right hand. At that moment, the infant's eyes close and she falls asleep, while the father continues talking, apparently totally unaware of the little miracle of specificity in time, place, and movement that had taken place in his arms.

Then, commenting on this interaction, Sander wonders:

> Are we looking at some principle of wholeness—that is, building on an underlying principle of specificity in time, place, and movement that joins directionalities between component systems—a joining that is necessary to construct coherent wholeness in a "system" that can be said to "live"?
>
> (2008, pp. 221–222)

It is fascinating to consider the possibility that such a dynamic—a *tendency* toward progressive fittedness—is also operating in the analyst/patient system. But what would such specificity look like in a moment, or more extended period, of analytic treatment with an adult? What would be required between an analyst and an adult patient with a history of developmental trauma to "join their directionalities" in such a way as to "construct coherent wholeness in a 'system' that can be said to 'live'"? Although Sander clearly believed the principles of development he had articulated were applicable to adult psychotherapy, he provided only limited, suggestive guidance in how to do this. He cited Schwaber's (1983) approach to analytic listening, and described a specific therapeutic intervention of Lyons-Ruth (2000), as two examples "of the use of specificity in recognition of state within the psychoanalytic framework" (Sander, 2002, 2008, p. 230).[3] I agree that Schwaber's model and Lyons-Ruth's vignette offer good examples of what the clinical application of Sander's thinking in adult analytic treatment might look like. But I don't think these examples alone do justice to the broader implications of his developmental model for clinical practice. He comes closer to capturing the fuller implications of his ideas in the following passage, which concerned living systems in general rather than the therapeutic dyad per se:

> I am asking, "Why not begin with uniqueness as a central principle in the organization of a living system?" I suggest further that specificity of recognition of that uniqueness—in an interactive system—is key to an organizing process based on constructing the essential specificity of connection between the components that is necessary to achieve the coherence or wholeness of the system required for the continuity of its life.
>
> (p. 226)

Sander had a knack for capturing large, complex ideas in felicitous, deceptively simple phrases or passages such as this succinct overview of his position. Applied to the analytic situation, he is saying that we begin with the central premise that every patient is a uniquely self-organizing system. He then equates the movement of the system (the patient) toward health with its movement toward a state of greater coherence or wholeness. This movement is made possible by an organizing process that evolves within the interactive system of patient and analyst through two key, interrelated processes: (1) progressive *specificity of recognition* of the patient in his uniqueness, and with that recognition, (2) progressive *specificity of connection*—i.e., specific forms of relatedness which implement the patient's recognized need of the moment. In a later passage Sander adds the dimensions of time and "recurrence": That is, the infant's or patient's state is constantly changing and evolving, calling for a recurring process of recognition and connection in repeated "moments of meeting."[4] He writes: "In as much as the developmental [or therapeutic] process is an ongoing flow of change, recognition of state itself must be an evolving process, constructing specificity of meeting in new configurations of increasing complexity as development [therapy] proceeds" (p. 228).

I find these organizing themes deeply resonant with my own understanding and vision of the analytic process. I would underline especially Sander's understanding that the achievement of fittedness or moments of meeting involves both *specificity of recognition* and *specificity of connection.* It is the ongoing combined experience of recognition and relational connection that provides the necessary organizing process for the patient to feel known and met in ways that motivate and facilitate his spontaneous movement toward greater wholeness—whatever wholeness might mean uniquely for a given patient at a given point in treatment.

Yet, as we all know, it is one thing to articulate elegant, abstract orienting principles and quite another to apply them in the messiness and uncertainties of actual moment-to-moment analytic work over years of real time with real, often profoundly traumatized, patients, given our own real limitations and vulnerabilities. The way that I make this link between orienting principles and clinical reality is through the intermediate area (Winnicott, 1971a) of psychoanalytic theories—broadly defined as all psychoanalytic (and neighboring) ideas and frames of reference that inform and constitute each of our analyzing subjectivities and capacities. Sander's ideas about fittedness and specificity cannot function as a stand-alone theory. Rather, like the concept of needed relationship, they are a set of meta-principles that relies on our evolving psychoanalytic theories for clinical implementation. Indeed, I view the emergence of new psychoanalytic theories as an expression of the meta-theoretical aim of achieving progressive fittedness with our patients as it operates at the level of the field of psychoanalysis as a whole. Our theories have emerged and evolved *for the purpose* of achieving greater fittedness—fittedness between what and how the analyst thinks, the actual nature of our patients' psyches and core problems, and the kinds of interventions needed to meet and transform those problems. The following represents my narrative for linking Sander's meta-theory of progressive fittedness and the emergence of actual needed relationships with our patients via the intermediate area of psychoanalytic theories, as they inform and constitute each analyst's analyzing subjectivity.

Clinical complexity and the analyst's analyzing subjectivity

Contemporary analytic theorists beginning with Winnicott (1965) have alerted us to the degree to which patient and analyst, like mother and baby, form an intersubjective system (e.g., Galatzer-Levy, 1978, 2002; Ogden, 1994; Stolorow, 1997a, b; Ghent, 2002; Beebe & Lachmann, 2002, 2014; Coburn, 2002, 2014; Seligman, 2005; Sander, 2008; Marks-Tarlow, 2008, 2011; Boston Change Process Study Group, 2010). The analytic process is in some ways analogous to successful problem-solving and interactive regulation between a caregiver and baby. Yet, it is also far more complex because it is a system competence (Sander, 1995) that must be responsive to the patient's history of relational trauma and system-*incompetence*, and the patient's complex psychological organization growing out of that history, as these now constitute and drive the patient's struggles. Because developmentally traumatized patients have grown up in situations that were decidedly *unfitted* to their early needs, their relational expectancies (transferences) and character adaptations incline them to be suspicious of, unpracticed in, resistant to, and even destructive of, the natural collaborative tendency observed in Sander's father-daughter video clip. *Thus analytic collaboration and fittedness must begin by meeting patients in spaces where being met is an alien, distrusted experience, which patients may misread, avoid, negate, or attack even as they unconsciously long for and seek it.* Analytic patients' distrustful, terrified, fragmented, deadened, overwhelmed, dysregulated, somaticized, disorganized, dissociated, colonized, and otherwise turbulent mental states (which are always embedded in, reactive to, and emergent from the ongoing analytic interaction) can only be transformed through systemic processes wherein the analyst learns through complex ongoing feedback at all levels of processing how to understand and respond to (meet) these states in increasingly individualized and nuanced ways. Moreover, leaps in analytic system competence often emerge from some form of enacted "incompetence" (Russell, 1998, 2006). Inevitably, there is trial and error, disruption and repair, negation and recognition, enactment and emergence from enactment, confusion or uncertainty and illumination, as the system gropes toward greater fittedness, specificity of recognition, mutual recognition, and hence greater system competence.

The implication of all of these clinical vicissitudes is that the analytic equivalent to what a good enough mother or father does naturally with a baby or young child in recurrent moments of meeting requires a high degree of *complexity in the analyst's subjectivity-as-analyst* (conscious, implicit, and unconscious), and in the observational, processing, intuitive, interpretive, and relational capacities that derive from and express that subjective complexity. If there could be said to be a *tendency* toward mutual regulation and fittedness between a patient and analyst comparable to that between a parent and young child, *the patient's job in that collaboration is to communicate through all means available* (free association and verbal communication generally, bodily states and communications, dreams, symptoms, transference, emergent and reactive mental states and moods, implicit/enactive behaviors, projective identifications, etc.) *the nature and "feeling" of what's wrong and in need of transformation, or what is underdeveloped and in need of developmental support.*

Drawing on Bion's (1962) concept of container/contained,[5] we could think of the patient's total communication to the analyst as the contained. The complexity of the contained (the patient's problems and struggles and how they manifest in the analytic interaction) requires at least comparable, and probably much greater, complexity in the analyst's receptive, processing, analyzing, and relational capacities in order for the analyst (and the analytic process) to function effectively as a container—that is, to be able to progressively grasp (consciously and intuitively) the complexities of the patient's conscious and unconscious communications, and thereby be able to meet the patient in successive approximations to, and negotiations of, relational fittedness. By "grasp" I don't mean primarily to understand the patient in an intellectual sense (although we *are seeking* to do this as a necessary component of our skills), I mean grasp in *the operational sense of being able to sense what to do next* based on one's total apprehension and processing of what is going on in the patient, the interaction (conscious and unconscious), and the field. From the analyst's standpoint, every analytic moment is an occasion for mindful engagement, where science and art meet and moment-to-moment, essentially creative, always-fateful choices need to be made in the service of facilitating the patient's movement toward his largely implicit and unformulated developmental aims.

Interestingly, as Lyons-Ruth (1999) has summarized them, the parenting qualities that have emerged as optimal for positive long-term developmental outcomes in the cognitive development, attachment, and infant-caregiver observation literatures sound strikingly similar to the analytic capacities I am highlighting as optimal for the achievement of progressive fittedness with adult patients:

> Developmental research on attachment relationships has also documented the features of developmental dialogue that are associated with flexibility and resilience in the child's later development. The convergence across studies and across different research traditions is unmistakable. Developmental communication systems that are open to the entire array of affective communications (e.g., Ainsworth et al., 1978); that include both participants' initiatives in a balanced, mutually regulated dialogue (Baldwin, Cold, and Baldwin, 1982); that are characterized by active negotiation and repairing of miscues, misunderstandings, and conflicts of interest (Tronick, 1989; Crockenberg, and Litman, 1990); and that are actively scaffolded by the developmentally more advantaged partner toward more flexible and inclusive forms (e.g., Wood, Bruner, and Ross, 1976) are associated with positive developmental outcomes for the child. These outcomes include affectively positive interpersonal relationships and enactive procedural models for conducting relationships that are coherent, integrated, flexible, and open to new information (see Bretherton, 1988, for review of this literature).
> (p. 583)

The point I am making is that providing the equivalent of these parenting capacities in the adult analytic context requires a complexity of grasp even greater than that required for good enough parenting.

The theoretical universe

What do I mean by the necessary complexity in the analyst's analyzing subjectivity, and how is it achieved? The common word for this subjective complexity is *wisdom*—a special kind of *analytic wisdom* that each analytic therapist develops uniquely according to her own personal aesthetic or idiom as an analyst, including her idiom of selecting, synthesizing, and reinventing psychoanalytic theories as she improvises in every session with every patient (Gabbard & Ogden, 2009). Of course, analytic wisdom is inseparable from whatever wisdom the analyst has derived from her life experience and clinical experience, but I am focusing here on the wisdom attained from the analyst's immersion in the universe of psychoanalytic ideas.

Different contemporary analytic authors have taken different positions regarding the scope of the theoretical universe from which they draw, and which, by implication, they regard as sufficient or optimal for analytic work. Some, like Mitchell (1988, 1993, 1997, 2000), find value in, and explicitly draw upon, the thinking of many theorists, old and new—indeed, believe that such integration is necessary because each major theorist offers important strands in the tapestry of analytic understanding. Bollas (1989) argued similarly, but couched in terms of patients' needs for their analysts to serve multiple functions:

> From my point of view, the contemporary analyst's task is to understand the many schools of analytic thought, as each represents a specific analytic function that needs inclusion in the psychoanalytic field . . . **The psychoanalyst is an object performing multiple functions . . . according to the clinical requirements of the analysand.** If the analyst can free himself from any freezing of his potential multiple functioning, then he can present the analysand with more usable objects within the analytic space and thereby avail the true self of more possibilities for the movement through an object as a fulfillment of its destiny.
>
> (1989, p. 100, bold in the original text)

Other contemporary theorists, for example Stolorow (e.g., Stolorow & Atwood, 1992), are at the other extreme. With the exception of Kohut, he and his co-authors for the most part repudiated earlier psychoanalytic theorists as misguided compared with their own epistemological and theoretical positions. And there is a third group of theorists somewhere in between. Ogden (1994, 2005, 2009) and Eigen (1981, 1996), for example, have tended to draw heavily on the work of a select few—primarily Freud, Klein, Bion, Winnicott, and Lacan—in their particular integrations.

Ogden (2005, 2009), like Bollas, has explicitly articulated his philosophy regarding the use of analytic theories. He cites Bion's (1962, p. 86) concept of "binocular vision," which argues for the need for multiple vantage points or vertices in the analyst's capacity to think about and process clinical interaction: "Viewing reality from multiple vantage points allows each vertex (each way of viewing reality) to enter into a mutually mutative conversation with other ways of seeing/knowing/experiencing" (2009, p. 96). As an example of this, Ogden (2005, Chap. 7) describes his binocular use of Winnicott's holding and Bion's container/contained functions: "Winnicott's holding and Bion's container/contained represent different analytic vertices from which to view the same analytic experience . . . Together they afford 'stereoscopic' depth to the understanding of the emotional experiences that occur in the analytic setting" (p. 108). At the same time, Ogden (2009, p. 90) also quotes Bion as saying: "Psycho-analytic virtue lies not in the number of theories the analyst can command but the minimum number with which he can meet any contingency he is likely to meet" (1962, p. 88).

My own approach, more like Mitchell's and Bollas's, tends to be broadly integrative of many theories and frames of reference—many potential vertices. Thus, while I agree with Ogden's (and Bion's) first principle regarding the need for binocular vision, I disagree with the second. From my perspective, the more of the total universe of psychoanalytic ideas an analytic therapist is able to command, the more potentially powerful is her capacity for binocular vision. My full thinking here would take us too far afield of the central themes in this chapter, but is a major focus in Chapter 2. Mainly, it has to do with the rapidly expanding universe of psychoanalytic theories and frames of reference, their increasing complexity, and the complexity of the interactions among them. (See also S. Stern, 2009a, b for a fuller elaboration of these ideas.[6])

Psychoanalytic healing

I have, in the previous two sections, described some of the complexity of the analyst's analyzing subjectivity necessary to meet relationally traumatized patients in ways that are analogous to Sander's father-daughter moment of meeting captured on video. But all of this cognitive and relational complexity, whether explicit or implicit, theoretically based or intuitive and improvisational, is not sufficient for achieving the "miraculous . . . joining of directionalities" Sander finds in this video sequence. The transcendent, primary, element left out of my formulations so far is the *love (and capacity to love)* this father obviously had in relation to his daughter (and vice versa, at a very different developmental level). The "miracle of specificity of time, place, and movement" we observe can only be comprehended in the context of the father's love for his daughter. If human development relies on love as the necessary motivator and guide for achieving progressive specificity of recognition and the meeting of relational needs, what are the implications for psychoanalytic treatment?

This question immediately brings to mind the idea of analytic love, which a number of relational authors, myself included, have been trying to define (Frankel, 1993; Davies, 1994; Bach, 2006; Fosshage, 2007; Mendelsohn,

2007; J.H. Slavin, 2007; Hoffman, 2009; S. Stern, 2011; Shaw, 2014). While the word love does, I believe, have its place in the analytic setting, it is tricky because, for the word to have any useful meaning, it has to be seen as a state that *develops* over time as a function of the deepening analytic relationship, as opposed to the more automatic and unconditional love that exists between a good-enough parent and infant. I say "more" because it can take time for some good-enough parents to feel fully attached to and unconditionally "in love with" their newborn children; and some analytic couples do experience the equivalent of love at first sight. Moreover, even if we can say that we develop a kind of attachment to, and love for, many of our patients, there is a necessary asymmetrical imbalance between the dependency and love our patients feel toward us, and that which we feel toward them. Moreover, it is impossible to separate the real love we have for our patients (and they for us) from the vicissitudes of transference and countertransference as these evolve over time. Indeed, the question of what is real vs. transference-countertransference in our relations with our patients is one of those Winnicottian paradoxes that probably is best left unresolved. In short, while analytic love exists and is, in my view, a crucial part of the therapeutic equation, in the analytic context it is more dependent than independent variable.

So, if love is not the answer, what is? It seems to me that *the impulse and capacity to heal psychoanalytically* is the analytic equivalent to a parent's impulse and capacity to love her or his child unconditionally and skillfully.[7] If unconditional love is the independent variable in good-enough parenting, the impulse or passion to heal our patients is the independent variable in psychoanalysis. It is the love of healing rather than the love of our patients per se that is our deepest, most fundamental motivation. Yet, there are paradoxes here, too, because the fullest psychoanalytic healing tends to occur in analytic dyads where analytic love *does develop* in a deep and unique way. I have noticed over the years that the experiences of healing and love are closely related, interdependent, and bi-directional, but that the patient's experience of feeling healed seems to be primary. If a patient feels deeply, and newly, understood and helped in some significant way, he more or less automatically (even if still ambivalently) feels more love (or at least trust) in relation to the analyst. That deepening of trust enables patients to be more emotionally vulnerable and expressive, which in turn evokes deepening love and trust in the analyst. Conversely, a patient may feel loved by his analyst, but if there is a failure in the experience of being truly helped, that love will not be experienced as therapeutic; indeed, it may well feel more like a repetition of parents who believed they felt love for their child without ever being able to recognize who the child they claimed to love actually was.

If there is a failure of analytic love to develop in treatments that are helpful, or if it existed but was subsequently lost, these are signs of problematic enactments—often repetitions of the unloving conditions of the patient's early relational milieu—that need to be understood and worked through in order for the fullest possible healing to occur. At the other extreme, if the analyst "loves too much"—if love seems to supersede or become equated with the healing process or the essential healing agent—that can also be a sign of a problematic (even potentially dangerous) enactment in need of analytic deconstruction. Because of the delicate, dynamically complex, and contingent nature of the development of analytic love, it needs to be underwritten by a more fundamental and unshakable commitment to psychoanalytic healing, which is operative even when (actually, especially when) feelings of love are not present or are still shaky. While many of the authors cited at the beginning of this section have offered definitions of analytic love that provide useful guidance, in my experience analytic love develops uniquely in each case, taking its form from the particular chemistry of the analytic pair and the cross-currents of love, fear, and negation that are central in each patient's lifelong struggles. In this sense, analytic love is *emergent* from the analytic couple's intersubjective engagement with the patient's (and, of course in the background, the analyst's) struggles and capacities in relation to love.

The *capacity* to heal psychoanalytically *develops* over a lifetime of immersion in psychoanalytic training, theory, and clinical experience. However, the *impulse* to heal psychoanalytically probably precedes psychoanalytic education; is operative throughout every psychoanalytic treatment from beginning to end; and, in conjunction with all we have learned from education, theory and practice, is what carries us through and motivates us to solve the many profound difficulties we can encounter in our efforts to achieve progressive fittedness with our patients. It does seem to me to be a form of love, but more a love of the unique intersubjective healing process with each patient, which ultimately requires unique forms of analytic love.

Thus I believe analytic clinicians' good-enough functioning must begin with a primary passion for and dedication to psychoanalytic healing—not in an abstract, idealized, grandiose, or fanatical way, but in the sense of loving the messy, often disturbing and preoccupying, but profoundly engaging and ultimately rewarding challenges involved in learning how to understand, be with, and truly help the "suffering strangers" (Orange, 2011) who become our patients. Beginning with Freud's (1915a) denunciation of Ferenczi's "*furor sanandi*" (passion or "rage" for healing) as a form of "fanaticism," a tradition has evolved in psychoanalysis of viewing therapeutic zeal as a misguided, if not neurotically driven, obstacle to the mental operations involved in coming to understand, and thus ultimately truly help, our patients. Bion (1970) echoed Freud's sentiment in his own disparagement of the need or "desire" to help, again as an interference with the radical, undirected openness and receptivity he believed necessary for the apprehension of the patient's psychic reality.

I understand the wisdom in Freud's and Bion's sentiments, but only as part of a complex paradoxical tension that any good analytic therapist must hold. For many if not all of us, our passion to heal has unconscious roots in needs to heal ourselves and/or the damaged familial figures of our childhoods—needs that can readily transfer to adult relational contexts with significant others, especially our relationships with our patients. This transferred need to heal is not all bad in as much as it fuels our impulse or passion to heal. But a need to heal and a passion to heal are not the same thing, which is how I hear both Freud's and Bion's cautionary advice. We get into trouble to the degree that we *need* to heal or help our patients, both because such a need constitutes a toxic impingement on a patient and because it interferes with the conscious and unconscious freedom the analyst requires to be able to apprehend, process, and respond in truly attuned and helpful ways to all that is occurring intersubjectively in the analytic field. Within the contemporary relational sensibility, this kind of passion would be understood as an enactment of some kind.

Yet, it seems disingenuous for our most prolific theoretical geniuses, who have devoted their entire lives to developing, continuously reworking, and teaching their understandings of how best to think about and help analytic patients, to act as if they are not possessed of a passion to heal psychoanalytically. The very insight that the desire to heal can seriously interfere with the analyst's optimal analyzing subjectivity, is itself motivated by the desire to heal. To say that an analytic clinician should eschew the passion to heal psychoanalytically seems no less absurd than telling parents they should eschew their passion to facilitate the best possible developmental outcomes for their children. Just as good-enough parents are passionate about really figuring out who their children are and what they need, psychoanalysts' necessary passion to heal is similarly oriented to figuring out who each of their patients is (specificity of recognition), and how best to help them, given the tools at hand (specificity of connection). Just as a mother's primary, unconditional love is what motivates and sustains her "live adaptation to her infant's needs" (Winnicott, 1965, p. 54), it is the analyst's passion to heal that motivates and sustains her live adaptation to her patient's needs.

In summary, it is in the context of treatments where the impulse and capacity to heal psychoanalytically are operative that an *intersubjective tendency toward progressive fittedness* becomes a plausible therapeutic factor.

Clinical example: Linda and me

Before launching into the specifics of my first extended case example I want to say that, because of the non-linear complexity of the processes I'm attempting to describe, the clinical narrative itself is less linear and more complex than those intended to demonstrate *particular* patient characteristics, qualities of analytic interaction, theoretical concepts, or therapeutic principles. As stated in Principle #9 (in the Introduction), I view the analytic relationship as a densely complex *transformational medium* with many elements in fluid interaction. The present example comes from a 9-year analytic treatment that I have written about twice before: once, at about the mid-point of treatment, in my 2009 paper, "The Dialectic of Empathy and Freedom" (Chapter 6 in this book); and a second time, looking back on the completed analysis, in my paper, "A 9-Year Analysis with a Connection-Resistant Patient" (S. Stern, 2014a). In both of those papers the clinical narratives are more linear and straightforward. Here, by contrast, because I am trying to capture the non-linear evolution of certain complex elements over time, the narrative circles around on itself in various ways and may require multiple readings for this complex moving picture to come fully into focus. Some of the elements I highlight are my complex therapeutic stance with Linda, the changes in that stance over time, the complex nature of the experience of time in our treatment, and the unique language and quality of each party's voice as these evolved over time.[8]

Time is a potentially complex factor in the two participants' experiences of the relationship as it unfolds. (See also Baranger & Baranger, 1961–1962/2009; Loewald, 1980; Model, 1993.) The needed relationship in a particular treatment develops cumulatively over time into discernable interaction patterns, processes, and phenomena, and these exert influence in the present moment of analytic interaction in the sense that all that occurs in the present moment grows out of all that has come before (Marks-Tarlow, 2008). Moreover, both the patient's and analyst's experience of each other in the present moment are not only reactions to what is happening now, but rather what is happening now *in light of* all that has come before. This is a dimension of needed relationships that tends not to be emphasized in clinical papers in which a particular theoretical or technical principle is illustrated with a dramatic vignette of a clinical interaction or sequence of interactions during a session or over the course of several sessions.

* * *

Linda, a successfully married woman in her 50s with a certain degree of psychological sophistication that had come from years of prior therapy of various kinds, was able, in our first meeting, to articulate some of what she hoped for in coming to a psychoanalyst. She said she needed a therapist who could "hold my feet to the fire," given that she could be "slippery" and "disappear from people." She said further that she hoped to learn "to be able to express disappointment and anger, to say clearly what I want, to feel vulnerable and connected." Linda's self-characterization was quickly borne out. My experience of her early in the analysis, confirmed by her own reported experience as well, was that when she was present she was fully, if anxiously, engaged, and engaging. But she also "disappeared" frequently, both from one session to the next, and by taking long breaks for international travel and therapeutic group experiences of various kinds. When she would return it was as if I hadn't existed for her and we were starting all over again, almost as strangers.

Looking back, if I had to say in a nutshell what the crux of the problem was for Linda and me, it was that the kind of deep relational connection—call it regression to dependence, surrender, or, in self-psychological parlance, a fully engaged selfobject transference—which I believed was necessary for the kinds of changes Linda was seeking in therapy, represented for her a toxic, dreaded, self-endangering merger, which she made clear she could and would never allow. The reason for this extreme allergy to dependency, we both came to understand, grew out of her childhood relationship with her mother wherein any merger or surrender meant to be taken over by the mother's needs and expectations, and to completely lose her self within a deadened and deadening intersubjective force field.[9]

Despite this understanding, the rudiments of which became clear very early on, I engaged in a years-long struggle with Linda around the half-in/half-out quality of her participation in the analysis, a struggle that, in retrospect, both she and I regarded as having been difficult but important, even essential, in helping her engage sufficiently to derive the profound benefits from our work that she did. There were many reasons I chose to pursue Linda regarding her absences, but one of the main ones (aside from my subjective feeling that her absences were compromising the engagement and development of an analytic process) was her all-but-complete dissociation/repression of long-standing feelings of sadness and rage, and a frightening sense she often had of drifting into inner darkness, aloneness, emptiness, and depression. If she found herself approaching any of these feelings in a session, she would immediately shut them down either with a sudden headache, an overwhelming sense of fatigue and wanting to go to sleep, or a strong urge to leave the session and go home. The way that I think about these things, I believed that in order for Linda to begin to tolerate these feelings she and I would need to develop a deeper emotional connection than was possible given the frequency of her disruptive absences, which could last 3 or 4 weeks at a time. My confrontations around this issue paid off in the sense that Linda was persuaded to commit to *some* long periods of increased session frequency with fewer and shorter vacation breaks. And, as I had hoped, these periods of more intensive involvement did result in a progressively deeper, more trusting connection between us, a great deal of productive analytic work across various life and intrapsychic domains, and an increasing capacity on Linda's part to feel her feelings. However, the sense that Linda was always keeping one foot out the door—always holding out the possibility that she could quit at any time—remained a feature of the treatment from beginning to end.

The following contextualized notes from early in our fifth year of work give the flavor of our interactions around the issue of her engagement through much of the analysis. They are from a period when I found myself feeling irritated because Linda had both cut back from 3 to 2 sessions per week (before I thought it wise to do so) and was either late for or missing even more sessions than usual. She was complaining of

> " . . . feeling adrift, in a fog," as if to say, "Why isn't this analysis helping me more?" I persisted with my belief that it was related to her attendance. I said I felt like a school principal telling a student: "You have to come to school every day to learn." Later that month she said she felt love from me at 3 times a week, but that I got angry and withdrew at 2 times. I asked: "Couldn't my anger be out of love?" . . . Two months later she returned from a 3-week trip and said that, for the first time, she had felt connected to me during it. I was there for her in the world. Previously, she had always reported not having thought of me at all during her absences—I essentially hadn't existed. This made me happy on many levels, which I expressed, but I also argued again for resuming 3 times a week, and, surprisingly, she now agreed! In the next session she reported a dream of *getting free of something (like a box) and falling upside down through space.* She feels therapy is helping her get free of something: her inner boxes. I responded that we weave connection out of disconnection. She liked that image. A month later she reported being in a good place, less anxious, and feeling it's connected to coming 3 times again.
>
> (S. Stern, 2014a, p. 188)

Note, in this example, that my interventions were aimed at, and held, the relationship on different time scales simultaneously. I was responding to what was happening in the present moment; at the same time, *à la* Loewald, I was holding the relationship in its long-term temporal dimension and experiencing the present moment as a point on a trajectory that incorporated both our already-multi-year experience with each other, and our potential future—a future I was nudging us toward.

Finally, there came a (tipping) point, relatively late in the analysis, when I started to become both more resigned to and accepting of Linda's way of being in analysis. I gradually surrendered (Ghent, 1990) to her need to control and limit our connection, rather than continuing to hold out for what might be. As I characterized it in my 2014 paper, my new attitude was: "When she comes she comes; what she does, she does; what she feels, she feels" (2014a, p. 189). This gradual act of surrender had a dramatic effect in that it led to a *mutual* surrender and greater mutual acceptance of our different subjectivities. Prior to this shift, it had been as if two implicit theories of therapeutic action had been competing within the potential space of my analytic subjectivity: (1) the belief that Linda needed to regress into a greater dependence and state of un-integration in order to be open to a new experience of relatedness (and hence a new experience of self) at the deepest levels—an idea I attribute mainly to Winnicott (1954); and (2) the belief that I needed to attune to, empathize with, and meet Linda exactly where she was, with no need or "desire" on my part except to recognize and perhaps (interpretively) name her emotional truth of the moment—an idea that, for me, comes from many sources but especially Bion (1967, 1970). These two theories existed in what I felt to be a necessary dialectical tension for much of the analysis, until finally a shift occurred (which was less a decision than a surrender) and the second theory assumed primacy.

The experience of time

A complex experience of the relationship as it existed in time played a significant role in both the early and late phases of the analysis. In the early phase, while trying to remain fully present to our interaction in the here-and-now, fully accepting of Linda as she was, and focused on understanding her, I was also nudging her toward a potential engagement, with an implied vision of what was possible in her, and our, futures—a variation on a developmental function (envisioning a patient's future) Loewald (1960) viewed as crucial to analytic needed relationships. Linda could not do this for herself because of the toxicity and paranoid anxieties associated with asymmetrical forms of dependency or surrender. Left to her own instincts, she would have continued to "disappear from people" with no change in the relational permeability, self-consolidation, and sense of aliveness she hoped for from the analysis. I had to perform the function of "holding her feet to the fire" (in tolerable doses), which I did mainly by respecting her present self while confronting her with the developmental requirements of the future self she hoped to become. This complex function of holding her situation on different time scales—an aspect of Winnicott's holding function (Winnicott, 1956; Ogden, 2005, Chap. 7)—became the vehicle through which she became able, slowly, to take the risks necessary to move toward her desired future.

In the late phase, after I had let go of this kind of confrontation and struggle, Linda's experience of me and our relationship shifted to a point where she could articulate that one of *her* remaining goals in treatment was "being able to internalize me enough so that she could function on her own without plunging into her dreaded state of aimless drifting, emptiness and darkness" (S. Stern, 2014a, p. 190). We both understood that accomplishing this would depend on a level of connectedness that required sufficient continuity in our meetings. She began another session playfully asking: "Will you be my mother?" (p. 189)—an idea which, in any form, would have been anathema to her throughout most of our time together. The greater freedom, intimacy, and surrender embodied in these statements clearly reflected Linda's experience of *my* surrender to her. But, I would argue, both of our experiences of surrender had the therapeutic power they did only in the temporal context of the years-long struggle that had preceded them. It was the *shift* in our transference-countertransference field, reflecting *my* capacity and willingness to change as an adaptation to her needs (Winnicott, 1965; Slavin and Kriegman, 1998), and, in response, *her* ability and willingness to change as well, which carried the therapeutic action and (in part) constituted the needed relationship in the later phase.

Our language and voices

In addition to illustrating the role and complexity of the experience of time in Linda's and my relationship, the above session notes also illustrate the complexity embodied in our *co-created language* and *voices with each other*. As is often the case in psychoanalysis, the themes and aims Linda had articulated in our first session played out in the treatment from beginning to end. One of the ways they were enacted was in Linda's and my unique language as it developed over time—a language I would characterize as one of *shared power*. *I* expressed power in my confrontations around Linda's engagement and commitment (thereby "holding her feet to the fire"), but tried to do so in a way that was primarily self-expressive and concerned rather than controlling—a critical difference for Linda, who had had a very controlling, unempathic mother. At the same time, Linda exercised *her* power in her increasing freedom to say exactly how she felt about me and how I was relating to her, becoming increasingly confident over time that I valued, and did not feel threatened (for the most part) by, her directness. This also was a needed new experience for Linda.

So, there was a complex dance going on around issues of power, control, and connection wherein power experienced as non-controlling and loving led, slowly and fitfully, both to a deepening connection between us and a developing sense of confidence, strength, and agency on Linda's part.

Yet, I would go further and say that my voice was even more complex than how I have characterized it thus far, and that this further complexity captures more fully the nuances of our evolved fittedness. Even as I said things like "I feel like a school principal . . . " and "Couldn't my anger be out of love?" there was a kind of space around these statements expressed in the quality or tone of my voice. Not consistently, but mostly, and more so as time went on, my tone conveyed, implicitly, that it wasn't that I *needed* Linda to change; I *wanted* her to change as part of a larger feeling of acceptance and the unique love that had formed between us. I know that Linda (mostly) heard this in my voice, even as we struggled seemingly against each other. I think there was also a paradoxical quality of *trying to influence Linda at the same time that I was letting things unfold.* To use Grossmark's (2012a) felicitous phrase, I was going with "the flow of enactive engagement," but part of that flow was my emergent, spontaneous efforts to advocate for what I believed would help. Thus even as I was exerting a kind of power, I was holding these initiatives lightly with a feeling of space around them—holding them (to paraphrase Winnicott, 1971a) as *inter*subjective objects, offered for Linda's potential, creative/destructive use and as a form of serious play unique to our co-created idiom. Thus she could say: "I felt love from you at 3 times a week, but you got angry and withdrew at 2 times." And I could reply without skipping a beat: "Couldn't my anger be out of love?"

* * *

To circle back around, in this case example the unique ways in which Linda's and my complex experiences of our power struggle as it existed in (and changed over) time, and the complex quality of our shared language and voices as these also evolved over time, illustrate the complexity of the analyst's subjectivity necessary to meet the unique complexity of the patient's subjectivity in the fitful movement of the dyad toward the achievement of progressive fittedness—i.e., the conditions necessary for the patient's growth and transformation. Of course, these were only two elements in the total complexity of our relationship as it evolved over time. Even in these brief excerpts one could point to any number of other concurrent elements, for example: our transference/countertransference dynamics and their meaning in terms of each of our internal object worlds (Cooper, 2014), attachment histories (Wallin, 2014), and projective identifications (Ogden, 1986, 1994; Tansey & Burke, 1989); or the erotic implications of Linda's and my power struggle and how it played out. But one of my points in using this example was to dramatize how Linda's and my uniquely improvised relationship is not reducible to any of these individual frames of reference. While they are all "in there," the unique specifics of our relationship were primarily patient- rather than theory-driven, and represented a complex amalgam of many factors operating simultaneously over time.

Enactment and intentionality

What about the role of enactment in Linda's analysis? The two discussants of my paper about Linda's 9-year analysis (Orange, 2014; Wallin, 2014) each found evidence of problematic enactments in the narrative, but different enactments related to each of their different orientations and interests. Orange (2014) perceived that my guiding theory (according to which Linda needed to surrender more to the process in order to achieve her therapeutic/developmental aim of being able to feel more vulnerable and connected) was causing me to pressure her in ways that mainly provoked and perpetuated her resistance. Wallin (2014), on the other hand, thought that I failed to recognize how my own attachment history was affecting my experience of Linda, and was therefore inadvertently constricting my participation and causing me to be overly controlling with her.

I can readily acknowledge that both of these perceptive discussants saw things that were present in my engagement with Linda and likely, at times, fueled the very resistance that I was seeking to engage and moderate. But my own sense, and ultimately Linda's as well, was that my confrontations were necessary and did more good than harm.[10, 11] These observations and my reactions to them (S. Stern, 2014b) speak to the elusive, subjective, and complex nature of the interactions we call enactments. I would say I pursued Linda in the way that I did *knowing* that I probably *was* enacting (consciously *and* unconsciously) both of the problems identified by the two discussants.

This kind of complexity points up an inherent messiness in the forms of engagement our patients sometimes need—a messiness not unlike that involved in parenting.

Final reflections: a tendency toward fittedness?

Listening to myself writing about this, I am disquieted by a quality in my argument that could easily sound self-valorizing. It may be an awkwardness inherent in writing about needed relationships and progressive fittedness that one has to focus on what seems to have worked. It also tilts the discourse more toward the intentional than the unintentional/unconscious/dissociated aspects of the analyst's participation—the latter being more prominent in the mainstream Relational literature. The humbling idea at the center of this perspective, however, is the mysterious possibility that the analyst does the kinds of things I did with Linda as part of a *tendency in the patient/analyst system to move toward progressive fittedness*. In other words, it was not just me but our co-created system of "directionalities," operating through both of our conscious and unconscious subjectivities and participation, which moved things in needed directions.

From this perspective, we could view Linda's early statement of her hopes for the treatment in our first meeting as her first gestures (Winnicott, 1960b), akin to the infant girl in Sander's video clip looking up at her father looking down at her, and beginning to raise her arm. Linda needed someone who could "hold my feet to the fire" because she was "slippery" and could "disappear from people," and at the same time help her "to be able to express disappointment and anger, to say clearly what I want, to feel vulnerable and connected"—a tall and complex order! In retrospect, it seems that somehow, over a 9-year period, we gradually co-created a relationship that did just that, and much more. In the end, just as the baby girl in Sander's video closed her eyes and fell asleep, Linda was able to relax enough into her newly internalized object relationship with me, and her much more confident and whole senses of self and agency, to be able to separate and leave.

Notes

1 We now know that Freud himself did not follow his own technical recommendations (Lipton, 1977; Lynn & Valliant, 1998; Baruch, 2014). Based on their study of 43 of Freud's cases seen between 1907 and 1939, Lynn and Valliant

concluded that "Freud's personal expressiveness and extra-analytic involvements invite consideration of each of these 43 analyses as a unique emotional and personal interaction between Freud and his analysand" (Lynn and Valliant, 1998, p. 170).

2 Orange (2012) has subsequently coined the term "developmental enactment" to differentiate this kind of "needed" engagement from the more problematic, "repetitive" forms.

3 The Boston Change Process Study Group (BCPSG), of which Sander was a member, incorporated several of his concepts into their groundbreaking formulations of the therapeutic process (D.N. Stern, et al., 1998; BCPSG, 2010). It is my view, however, that the group's synthesis departs in fundamental ways from Sander's holistic vision, and hence also from the integrative sensibility I present throughout this book. In particular, their bifurcation of analytic interaction into two allegedly separable dimensions (implicit/procedural vs. explicit/verbal/symbolic), and privileging one dimension (the implicit) *over* the other in their deconstruction of therapeutic action, moves in the opposite direction from Sander's project of understanding the mysterious processes through which human beings develop the senses of "coherent wholeness" (identity) and personal agency. See Chapter 5 for my full thinking about these issues.

4 Sander's use of the phrase "moments of meeting," unlike the Boston Change Process Study Group's later (D.N. Stern et al., 1998) use of the term to refer to infrequent, charged, dramatic analytic moments of attuned, authentic therapist responsiveness, is essentially synonymous with his concept of fittedness. It refers to the interaction between a baby and a good-enough mother in which the mother, *on an ongoing basis*, intuitively recognizes the infant's need or state of the moment and, in concert with the infant's implicit signaling, responds in ways that are specifically fitted to the infant's need or state, or its movement toward a coordinated task like breast-feeding. Sander underlines the fact that such moments of recognition and fittedness are "needed events," and that the reliable recurrence of such moments over time provides a needed foundation for the infant's development of basic trust, and ultimately a child's sense of agency and identity.

5 Bion's framing of *container/contained* as a single word seems similar in its implications to Sander's suggestion of an intersubjective *tendency* toward progressive fittedness.

6. My thinking about these issues is very much in keeping with Aron's (2009) and Aron & Starr's (2013) inclusive view and definition of psychoanalysis (S. Stern, 2009a, b).

7 "Skillful means" is a Buddhist term connoting both competence and wisdom.

8 Readers may find it helpful to return to this rendering of Linda's and my process after reading the more extended account in Chapter 6.

9 This paragraph was excerpted from S. Stern, 2014a (p. 181).

10 Ferro and Civitarese (2015) speak to the function of confrontation in a way close to my thinking with Linda: "Confrontation, then, is basically a useful instrument; however it is not so much specifically "psychoanalytic" as, in a broad sense, educational . . . that is, an appeal to common sense and observance of rules on occasion actually serves a deeper purpose of containment." (Kindle Edition, Chapter 7, "Mario": para. 3)

11 During a 1-year follow-up session, reflecting on our time together, Linda said that following *every* such confrontation, "even though I didn't like them, something shifted."

Chapter 2

Complexity made simple; simplicity made complex

The view of analytic needed relationships introduced in Chapter 1 reflects my perspective on the changing nature of psychoanalysis as a professional field, and on what qualifies a therapeutic relationship, or a given intervention, to be considered psychoanalytic (S. Stern, 2009a, b). Psychoanalysis as a field has, in my view, reached a point where it can no longer be defined by a particular theory, particular external frame criteria such as session frequency or the couch, or even a particular conception of the process. Not only have such conceptions become problematic because no two analytic schools of thought agree on them, our field has simply become too large and complex to fit into this kind of conceptual package. Rather, more like medicine or clinical psychology, I believe we need to redefine ourselves in terms of the human problems we address, and our *total* evolving field of inquiry and knowledge. (See also Aron, 2009.) The latter subsumes *all* of our major theories, and hundreds, if not thousands, of more circumscribed conceptual frames of reference pertaining to all aspects of the phenomena we study and treat—the nature of mind, the unconscious, development, psychopathology, the analyst's listening stance, transference and countertransference, the analytic process, therapeutic action and technique, and the social, ethical, and philosophical underpinnings of the analytic situation.

Until recently one could speak of psychoanalytic *pluralism* and, in our training programs, the teaching of *comparative psychoanalysis*, as terms for capturing the increasing complexity analysts face in both learning and using our major theoretical models. One could identify these models clearly, compare them on a variety of dimensions, and think about one's own analytic approach as either seeking to work within a given model, selectively incorporating aspects of different models into a personal synthesis, or simply using elements from different models in an eclectic, pragmatic, not-particularly-integrated way. Although we still think about our potential uses of different theories in these ways, I believe the theoretical field has become so complex that these old terms for conceptualizing our "relationship" to theory no longer capture the complexity of what is now involved in the processing of psychoanalytic theories and relating them to practice.

There are a number of dimensions to this increasingly complex task. First is the fact that we now have different kinds of theories that are not fully commensurable in a comparative sense. There are comprehensive theories, which, like Freud's various theories, provide a systematic matrix of concepts that address the nature of mind, development, psychopathology, the psychoanalytic situation, the psychoanalytic process, therapeutic action, and psychoanalytic transformation. Kohut's self psychology, in the later phases of his work (Kohut, 1977, 1984), falls in this category, as does Sullivan's (1953) interpersonal theory. At the other extreme are theories that focus on one or two of these elements—for example, Schwaber's (1983) approach to psychoanalytic listening (cited in Chapter 1).

I would include in this latter category the part-theories emanating from neighboring research fields, for example: contemporary attachment theory (Fonagy, 2001; Wallin, 2007; Lyons-Ruth & Jacobvitz, 2008; Slade, 2014); mentalization theory (Fonagy, et al., 2002; Bateman & Fonagy, 2016); and models emphasizing the implicit relational dimension of analytic interaction (D.N Stern, et al., 1998; Lyons-Ruth, et al., 1998; Boston Change Process Study Group, 2010; Beebe & Lachmann, 2002, 2014). These bodies of work and theory are exerting increasing influence on our understanding of both development and analytic interaction (Teicholz, 2015) but could not, I would argue, be employed as stand-alone theories. Rather, they must be combined with other psychoanalytic concepts to be useable. In some ways these research-based theories and frames of reference seem to be implicitly aiming to replace the more comprehensive developmental theories of Sullivan, Winnicott, Bion, Kohut, and others. Yet, these newer theories only cover certain dimensions of development, leaving large swaths of developmental territory under-theorized. The result is to leave practitioners with the increasingly complex task of somehow, on their own, integrating the findings and principles from these circumscribed, research-based theories and the more comprehensive narratives grounded in data from the psychoanalytic situation.

In addition to these differences in scope, there are also differences of *type*. For example, Hoffman's (1998) dialectical-constructivist vision of the psychoanalytic situation is a kind of meta-theory, much of which is potentially applicable regardless of an analyst's primary theoretical commitments. His ideas reflect his relational sensibility, but he focuses on certain existential and epistemological aspects of the psychoanalytic relationship, as well as dialectical tensions in the analytic interaction and the analyst's technical stance, which are superordinate to any particular theory and thus could potentially be integrated with a range of theories or schools of thought. However, to actually attempt such an integration of Hoffman's ideas with more classical (less relational) theories necessitates modifying the latter in complex ways.

Dialectical and paradoxical thinking also play central roles in both Winnicott's and Ogden's theoretical narratives. These trends in their thinking will be more fully referenced later in this chapter. Similar to Hoffman's dialectics, while these dimensions of their work arise from their more specific theoretical orientations, they transcend these contexts, as reflected in the frequency with which they are cited and integrated into the thinking of authors working across the full spectrum of psychoanalytic theories.

Yet, these problems of scope and type are only part of the new complexity. The complexity also results from the fact that, since the early 1980s, some of the most influential contemporary theories are not unitary theories in the sense that classical, Kleinian, interpersonal, or self-psychological theories were. They are really creative integrations, recontextualizations, and extensions of previous theories. Mitchell's (1988, 1993, 1997, 2000) relational-conflict theory is the paradigmatic example. Mitchell viewed one of his major contributions as bringing together existing concepts from diverse schools of thought into a new theoretical integration or context. He also introduced many new concepts such as his central metaphor of a "relational matrix" with both intrapsychic and interpersonal dimensions. But, at least as important as the concepts themselves was the style of theorizing within which they were generated. Mitchell, initially in collaboration with Greenberg (1983), undertook comprehensive reviews of previously existing theories and, to use one of his own metaphors, wove selected elements from them into a new tapestry. The word "selected" is important here. Mitchell was clear that he was rejecting certain elements of old theories—elements that were logically incompatible with the core assumptions of relational theory. But other concepts were retained and *recontextualized* within his new amalgamated relational theory. His (1988) reworking of the concept of, and therapeutic approach to, narcissism was a prime example, as was his redefinition of intrapsychic conflict.

The complexity grows when one recognizes that many other contemporary theorists do something similar to Mitchell, but each in her or his unique way. To name only a few of the most influential, Bollas, Ehrenberg, Aron, Ogden, Stolorow, and Benjamin all grounded their contributions in re-evaluations and re-contextualizations of earlier theories, each one selectively rejecting and incorporating different elements from these theories: each, in effect, establishing her or his own particular relationship to previous theories. Thus, when we read them and incorporate their thinking into our work, we are internalizing not just new theories but new complex relationships with earlier theories. And, each of their relationships to these earlier theories is unique and conflicts with that of the others, sometimes in fundamental ways. Stolorow and his associates thoroughly rejected the concept of projective identification (Stolorow, Orange, & Atwood, 1998), whereas Ogden (1994, 1997) continued to use it centrally in his work, but recontexualized within his concepts of the intersubjective analytic third and subjugating third. The task of relating theory to practice obviously is simplified if one chooses to follow one theorist or school above, or to the exclusion of, all others. If, however, one elects to remain open to the profusion of contemporary theories, and the recontextualization of earlier theories on which these new theories rest, one is faced with a task of enormous and ever increasing complexity as one attempts to incorporate this expanding field of ideas into one's work.

Finally, there is the special case of *complexity* or *non-linear dynamic systems theory*, which is in a category all of its own in that its proponents make claims for its being a paradigm-changing, superordinate meta-theory for psychoanalysis (e.g., Galatzer-Levy, 1978, 2002, 2009; Thelen & Smith, 1994; Stolorow, 1997a, b; Coburn, 2002, 2014; Ghent, 2002; Seligman, 2005; Harris, 2005; Marks-Tarlow, 2008, 2011; Boston Change Process Study Group, 2010). These authors have focused mainly on the analytic and mother-infant dyads as the systems of interest. The interactions of these dyads over time are shown, or at least interpreted, to reflect laws or properties comparable to those governing other complex biological and physical systems. Sander's (2008) concepts of specificity of recognition and progressive fittedness are grounded in a complex systems framework, as is much of my own thinking about needed analytic relationships.

The proponents of a complexity sensibility in psychoanalysis tend to remain vague, however, regarding the relationship between non-linear dynamic systems theory and the universe of psychoanalytic theories and frames of reference, which, of course, the therapists (usually themselves) in all of their clinical examples are employing. I doubt any of these authors believe that non-linear dynamic systems theory can function as a stand-alone framework for guiding analytic work. Indeed, many refer to ideas and principles, especially from relational theories, as moving in the same direction as, and thus implicitly supporting or validating, complexity theory concepts. What these authors (or at least their writings) fail to emphasize is that non-linear dynamic systems theory, as applied in an analytic context, has a *symbiotic* relationship with psychoanalytic theories. That is, complexity theory concepts can only be applied analytically in contexts where the therapist is also guided by concepts from psychoanalysis. It may be true—in fact, is true—that the adoption of a non-linear complexity perspective, like other paradigm-changing breakthroughs, alters and reorganizes an analyst's selective use, contextualization, and integration of psychoanalytic theories. But in order to become a psychoanalytically useable theory, it must "join up" with psychoanalytic theories in ways that further complexify the analyst's relationship to the contemporary universe of psychoanalytic theory.

A related area that remains vague in the complexity theory literature is the relationship between what is going on *within* the analyst's mind—her analyzing subjectivity—and the patterns or movement of interaction *between* patient and analyst that are presumably governed by the principles of complexity theory. The analytic dyad seems to me different from other complex systems (even other complex human systems such as caregiver-infant) in that the behavior of the analytic dyad as a system is so disproportionately influenced by the analyst's analyzing subjectivity and capacities. For example, if an analytic dyad is to shift out of a period of felt stuckness (in system theory terms, out of a rigid attractor state), it is the analyst's analyzing subjectivity that, most likely though not necessarily always, will have to generate processes that initiate such a shift. This is not to say that the analyst's analyzing subjectivity is not fully embedded in the complexity of the dyadic system and analytic field. Whatever the analyst says and does emerges from the infinitely complex intersubjective and field processes that situate the analyst's subjectivity. But it is nonetheless the analyst's responsibility to somehow operate within this infinitely complex system in ways that move the system in analytically productive directions. Indeed, learning about the workings of non-linear dynamic systems presumably becomes a feature of the analyst's analyzing subjectivity that makes such productive influence more likely! (See especially Coburn, 2014.) This fact renders the patient-analyst system particularly complex in ways that, in my view, have yet to be adequately addressed by authors in this area. My somewhat cumbersome solution is to posit a second complex dynamic system simultaneously at work: the extremely complex thinking and processing going on in the analyst's analyzing subjectivity on a moment-to-moment basis as she draws on all she knows while simultaneously interacting with and processing each patient's (and her own) subjectivity and behavior in the context of the analytic exchange and analytic field.

This understanding leaves open the question of what exactly the nature of the relationship is between the complex system of the dyad and the one going on in the analyst's mind. One of the reasons I am drawn to Sander's developmental principles and language is that they create a metaphorical bridge between the objective-descriptive perspective of complexity theory and the phenomenological perspective of an analytic therapist-at-work. Fittedness, for example, both describes a desired state of the system *and* evokes the phenomenological experience of participating in the self-organizing processes that lead to the achievement of this state. That is, we move fitfully toward progressive fittedness in part by way of the subjective feel of how well our current understanding and relational positioning fits with our own intuitive sense of what is needed, as well as with the patient's implicit communications regarding whether what we are saying and doing fits with *their* implicit sense of what they need. Only when the two are in relative alignment or harmony has a state of sufficient specificity or fittedness been achieved. Thus, through language that manages to be both scientific and poetic, Sander reimagines the non-linear dynamics of human, developmentally-purposed, dyadic systems as *inter-phenomenological dynamics* wherein the *objective* properties of the system are expressed through the evolving, emergent inter-*subjective* dynamics of the two system components (patient and analyst; parent and infant).

Heard in this way, Sander's language opens up potential links (a potential space) between complexity theory and psychoanalytic theories. For example, I find homologies between systems theory concepts and certain Bionian field theory concepts (Ogden, 1994; D.B Stern, 2013a, b; Ferro & Civitarese, 2013; Peltz & Goldberg, 2013). Viewing the patient-analyst dyad as a non-linear complex system moves in the same direction as viewing the dyad as existing within an analytic field or third, which is greater than the sum of its parts and whose operational laws or properties are not reducible to intersubjective dynamics alone. Integrating the contemporary Bionian and complexity perspectives yields a paradoxical understanding of the relationship between the complex system of the dyad and the one going on within the analyst's subjectivity: namely that *it is the analyst's job to "contain" the system that "contains" her.* I will return to a consideration of this paradox and its implications in Chapter 4. My point for now is that it is clear that the incorporation of complexity theory into our theoretical universe adds another layer of complexity to our contemporary relationship with psychoanalytic theories.

* * *

The concept of needed relationships, as I intend it, "floats" on this sea of complexity. Implicit in the concept is the understanding that the analyst's idiomatic, mostly implicit or preconscious use of existing ideas about psychoanalytic needed relationships (and psychoanalytic theories more generally) is itself a complex, evolving, dynamic system. Thus, a given intervention in a given moment represents the analyst's effort, based on the complexity of all that she knows, and the complexity of all that is going on intersubjectively in the present analytic moment, to do that which is needed to further the analytic process.

The yield of all of this conceptual complexity is, paradoxically, a kind of *simplicity*—an ever-improving capacity to respond to our patients in ways that, to invoke Sullivan, are "simply human," yet remain analytic, whatever that might mean in a given instance. From a fittedness perspective, advances in psychoanalytic theory and understanding, and their increasing complexity, bring us closer and closer to the live pulse of the clinical exchange and thus closer to being able to do the equivalent of what the father in Sander's brief video segment (quoted in Chapter 1) did with his infant daughter. I would actually say that this paradox is a defining characteristic of the analytic holding environment our patients need and expect from us. They need our simple humanity, but they also implicitly count on our complex grasp of both the nature of their struggles and the analytic process as it unfolds from moment to moment.

A crisis in my work with a patient, Suzanne, which came out of nowhere and proved to be a defining, transformational moment in the evolution of our analytic needed relationship, demonstrates this paradox in action.

Doing my job

The following sequence of events occurred about a year and a half into Suzanne's twice-a-week analytic treatment. A third party, a former friend of Suzanne's, had, without informing her, contacted me to invite me to become involved in a professional activity with her. Given my interests, it was something I would ordinarily have been strongly inclined to do. But because I remembered Suzanne having talked about this person as someone who had been a source of emotional distress in her life, I, with some trepidation, made the unusual decision to call and run this by her before answering the woman's request.

Suzanne was taken aback by my call, but as the reality sank in she became increasingly distressed. Feeling both guilty and embarrassed about having a problem with it, she said she wasn't sure how to advise me, but said how much she appreciated my calling to check it out with her. I suggested we schedule an extra session quickly to talk about the dilemma, and, despite our busy schedules, we found a time the next day to do so. I went into that session not sure what I would do because the activity I was being invited to participate in was not one I would automatically assume would interfere with Suzanne's analysis. However, it became clear during this special session that Suzanne felt so threatened by my having any relationship with this person that she felt it might seriously affect our work. I tried to explore the intensity of her feelings and anxieties in relation to this other person. She was able to say a few things, some of which I already knew, about how this former friend kept finding ways to enter her world and take things for herself, no matter what the collateral damage to Suzanne. But, from the obvious sense of dread and panic that overtook her as we spoke, I could tell this was not the time for such exploration and reflection. I could see that much as she wanted to be generous about it, she really would not be able to tolerate it if I entered into a relationship of any kind with this other person, even if I never spoke of it again.

Thus, whatever principle I might have invoked to justify treating the invitation as something separate from Suzanne's treatment, or something I shouldn't allow her to control, my decision became clear: I could not and would not work with the third party. With some inner difficulty on my part, given that I had hoped things might go the other way, we discussed together how I would communicate my decision to the former friend while protecting Suzanne's confidentiality. Suzanne remained in disbelief until I was able to report carrying out the plan, and stated emphatically that the issue was now resolved. Suzanne revealed at this point that she wasn't sure she would have continued in treatment had I not handled it the way I did.

This crisis proved to be transformative for Suzanne and for our relationship. In the immediate aftermath of this unusual sequence of events, Suzanne expressed embarrassed gratitude suffused with an unmistakable narcissistic glow. The crisis left her feeling a greater sense of confidence in me, and in herself, than she had previously. This is actually an understatement. Prior to this incident, although I would describe Suzanne's transference toward me as predominantly positive and idealizing, there was an underlying anxiety and distrust. I think she felt that I remained untested and that, in the crunch, under pressure from my own narcissistic needs, I would sell her out as both of her parents had done in different ways. It would either take the form of her revealing some hidden aspect of herself that I would find contemptible and deserving of rejection, or she would tempt me into some kind of dual relationship, as she had done with other male authority figures in the past. Either way, she assumed I would ultimately fail her, thus leaving her alone with her anxieties, outside the pale of the human community she longed to be a part of, and haunted by the cynical belief (Weiss, Sampson, et al., 1986) that no one on whom she might depend would ever come through for her and do their job in relation to her, whatever that might mean.

The understanding that, given her history, she was acutely sensitive to whether or not people were "doing their jobs" was an organizing theme that had grown out of our work during the first year and a half. My job was to perform my sacred function (Winnicott, 1971b) of being her analyst in a competent, dependable way, no matter what the pressures or tests I might encounter. I believe this is how my handling of our crisis resonated with Suzanne at the deepest levels. Although I knew most of this at the time that this emergency intruded itself, I would not say that I intentionally sought to provide a corrective emotional experience. I think the main thing I was conscious of was wanting to find a solution that would work for both of us. I decided that to do that I needed Suzanne to be involved so I could directly assess what was at stake. In doing so, my struggle became our struggle. Yet, the cost to her of being included in the end proved well worth the gain to me and us, which was that, having worked it through together, I could make the sacrifice without resentment.

In the weeks following, there was a new, palpable sense of calm (analogous, I would argue, to the baby girl in Sander's illustration of specificity falling asleep at the conclusion of the sequence with her father). A nervous vigilance was gone, and Suzanne's deeper trust freed her to bring more of herself into the open with much less anxiety that she might do or say something that could undo our relationship. And, amazingly to me, the shift lasted, throughout the duration of the 5-year treatment and beyond. It's not that there weren't ups and downs. There were, but we weathered these with the result that, overall, our connection strengthened. Suzanne's sense of calm, along with her ability to reflect on her previously unformulated early relational and emotional experience, with ongoing analytic work, continued to widen into all of the life domains (and their intrapsychic counterparts) in which she had struggled historically, including most centrally her relationship with her almost psychotically narcissistic mother. In analytic work following the crisis, we came to understand that the former friend who precipitated the crisis was heir to an intense maternal transference.

The complexity/simplicity dialectic

In one sense, someone (for example, someone unburdened by immersion in psychoanalytic theory) might say I did the simple human thing with Suzanne in this moment of crisis. Confronted with a conflict between a tempting professional involvement and the possible negative consequences to Suzanne and her treatment of my agreeing to participate, I did the reasonable thing: I bounced it off Suzanne, listened carefully to her reaction, then made what seemed to be the therapeutically wisest choice—not to pursue the involvement. It's all pretty straightforward—an ordinary example of human decency in the context of a therapeutic relationship. But in analysis few things are ever that simple (Baranger & Baranger, 1961–1962/2009), a cigar is rarely just a cigar, and this sequence of events between Suzanne and me was no exception.

We know that what occurred was not only a simple act of considerateness, for which Suzanne was appreciative; it was also therapeutically transformative. Something about this sequence of events consolidated Suzanne's trust in me, confidence in herself, and faith in our therapeutic process, and the question is: Why? What exactly happened here that made such a difference? Actually, to say that these events were in and of themselves transformative would be an oversimplification. They were only transformative in the context of an analytic relationship that had been evolving for a year and a half prior to this crisis and continued for several years beyond it. Even so, the events themselves dramatically changed things.

The choices I made were not only grounded in my ideas about human decency and thoughtfulness; they represented an extended moment of psychoanalytic improvisation made possible by my immersion (intellectually and experientially) in the history of ideas about psychoanalytic needed relationships. It's not that I had all of these consciously in mind as I navigated through the crisis. Ogden (2009), echoing Bion (1967, 1970), has suggested that the art of psychoanalytic improvisation requires: first the inculcation, then, paradoxically, the "forgetting" of the received body of knowledge and technique that constitutes our field of inquiry and clinical application. I'm not sure I would say, even paradoxically, that we forget what we have learned; rather, I think of it as a growing confidence or faith in our (increasingly complex) psychoanalytic instincts or intuition, which comes with intellectual and clinical immersion and mastery, and which in turn allows for greater freedom and spontaneity, and a humanness that is both simple and complex.

In order to give the flavor of the kind of implicit complexity that makes possible simply human psychoanalytic improvisations such as mine with Suzanne, I will deconstruct some of the psychoanalytic frames of reference that, in retrospect, must have informed my intervention. Much of this complexity has to do with changes in our understanding of the relationship between the *real*, the *transferential*, and the *symbolic* in the analytic relationship. Whereas, in traditional theory it was thought that keeping the analytic relationship relatively *unreal* (i.e., uncontaminated by intrusions of the analyst's real self) was ultimately what made possible the patient's capacity to engage and work through transference, to face and symbolize unconscious, drive-based, emotional experience, and thereby to grow psychologically, in contemporary relational theory it is recognized that the *realness* of the relationship, and real happenings in it, contribute powerfully to analytic growth and are part of what makes symbolization possible. The complexity in this statement resides mainly in the word *real* when used in a psychoanalytic context.

As a starting point for considering this complexity one can easily imagine that a traditional American analyst working 50 or 60 years ago would have handled the situation in exactly the opposite way from what I did and, ironically, probably would have considered *that* choice to be a relatively simple, straightforward one—indeed, perhaps not even a choice at all. Operating within the framework of American ego psychology, he would have made a sharp differentiation between the "real" and "transference" dimensions of the analytic relationship (Greenson, 1967). In that model, the real relationship was a given, but was seen as a kind of frame and not central to therapeutic action. Most likely, he would have seen the potential relationship with the third party as separate from the analytic relationship, might well have pursued it without saying anything to Suzanne, and if it came up later would have regarded it as an opportunity to work with Suzanne's largely pre-configured negative transference.

This binary between the real and the transferential began to be deconstructed with Gill's (1979, 1982a) realization that transference is always partly constructed from the real—the analyst's real qualities and the real interaction. It was further deconstructed by Hoffman's (1983) and Stolorow and Atwood's (1992) clarifications that both the patient and the analyst are always experiencing the other through the filters of their own subjectivities, histories, and organizing principles. In effect, the real is always, to some degree, transference and vice versa on both sides of the relationship. Moreover, in their constructivist, hermeneutic models, the now fully embedded analyst loses the ability to confidently and objectively differentiate between the real and the transferential (and especially between the real and the countertransferential). From these contemporary perspectives, regardless of how I decided to handle my crisis with Suzanne, those choices, sooner or later, would likely have had real impacts on our relationship, including the transference relationship. This understanding is both freeing and daunting in situations like the one I faced with Suzanne: freeing in that I was not overly concerned that taking the risks I did would *necessarily* be unanalytic or undermine our analytic process; daunting in that I was acutely aware that all of the options I could envision involved risks, and that how exactly I chose to handle the situation might well affect both our relationship and the analytic process going forward. Given the choices I did make, the realness of both my own participation and my enlistment of Suzanne's participation—especially the fact that, in plain view, I ended up making a personal, professional sacrifice in deference to her therapeutic needs—accrued positively not only to her experience of me as a decent human being but also as a new object in the transference.

Winnicott (1971a), coming from a very different theoretical tradition, introduced a perspective on the real that has reached far into contemporary thought: namely, his recognition of the paradox, similar to the paradox of a child's relationship to transitional objects, that what the patient makes of the analyst is always constructed from "what is there to be perceived" and what is subjectively created. In his words:

> For me [standard analysis] means communicating with the patient from the position in which the transference neurosis (or psychosis) puts me. In this position I have some of the characteristics of a transitional phenomenon, since although I represent the reality principle, and it is I who must keep an eye on the clock, I am nevertheless a subjective object for the patient.
>
> (1962, p. 166)

In this model the analytic relationship becomes a form of serious play whose power lies in the paradoxical mix-up of the real and the "as if." It is in this "intermediate" potential space where the real is both found and created, and where inside meets outside, that the capacity for symbol generation originates. From this perspective, the transformative power of my inclusion of Suzanne in my decision-making process arose not simply from my actions per se but from what she made of them creatively. One thing she made of them, which had already become a theme that we had identified, was that she experienced me here as *doing my job* in relation to her analytic needs. There is the further implication in Winnicott's (1969) vision that therapeutic action and psychological growth often result less from interpretations than from the experience of *living through something together* and *surviving*, whatever that might mean in a given instance. Clearly, that perspective applies here.

Winnicott's ideas about potential space, combined with elements from the Kleinian-Bionian tradition (and other non-psychoanalytic frames of reference) led to the emergence of various field theories such as the Barangers' (1961–1962/2009) analytic field and Ogden's (1994) analytic third. These models further complicate the relationship between the real and the transferential, and the real and the symbolic, by positing an unconsciously co-created intersubjective field within which each party's experience of the other (and self with other) is a product of this encompassing transference-countertransference matrix, which can only occur within an analytic frame. These models clarify that all experience within an analytic context is essentially and necessarily *ambiguous*—it is always what it is and something else, always real *and* transference or countertransference. Moreover, in these models, as in all contemporary relational theories of enactment, symbolization becomes possible from the analyst's capacity to be a full and real participant in the field, while also being able to reflectively process her experience through an internal dialectic between her individual analytic subjectivity and her subjectivity within the field or third (Ogden, 1994). From the perspective of these field theories, my choices and participation in this interaction were not simply expressions of my clinical subjectivity as a separate individual; they were shaped and prompted in part by the total transference-countertransference matrix that had been evolving. For example, the fact that I experienced this crisis as a conflict between my own desire and Suzanne's therapeutic needs was both real *and* an aspect of our unique transference-countertransference relationship. Again, it wasn't that I was consciously thinking about these field theories at the time; it's more that I had internalized them in a way that allowed me to abandon myself to the "flow of enactive engagement" (Grossmark, 2012a), trusting that whatever happened would likely, ultimately, be interpretable or at least useable in the service of opening up the analytic field as a therapeutic potential space.

Yet another relevant tributary, flowing from yet a different theoretical tradition, is Ehrenberg's (1992) model of working at "the intimate edge." One of her most subtle and important contributions was her recognition that the analyst has a real, lived relationship with the patient, albeit within a certain frame and role structure, and that therapeutic action involves the complex process of simultaneously living that relationship and carefully scrutinizing it as the foundation for symbolization and analytic growth. In her model the line between transference (or countertransference) and the real virtually disappears, and what matters is the close collaborative analytic attention paid to the emotionally real as it unfolds in the interaction of the subjectivities of both parties. I would say that it was in the nature of Suzanne's and my analytic alliance that we were able to both "live" this crisis and think about its possible meanings and implications even as we improvised, but especially in the weeks and months following.

In retrospect, perhaps the most transformative aspect of what happened is best captured by Ehrenberg's model, augmented by some of Davies' (1994, 2004) subsequent ideas about countertransference disclosure/exposure. Suzanne perceived that I was struggling between my own strong professional interests and doing what was best for her. The fact that she actually observed me assessing her needs and capacities in the situation, and then allowed that assessment to determine my decision despite my personal disappointment, was probably, more than anything else, what moved and impressed her. My choice was truly made at "the intimate edge" where my emotional reality and hers met in a conflict, which I resolved by deciding, based on my empathic assessment of her psychic reality, that at that particular analytic moment her reality took precedence. (See also Benjamin's, 2004, concept of a "moral third.") This was a new, needed experience of someone charged with her care doing their job in the crunch of conflicting needs.

At a different level of abstraction, Hoffman's (1998) various technical dialectics seem relevant to this encounter and were undoubtedly in the background as I made the choices I did. The dialectic between spontaneity and analytic ritual or discipline, and of mutuality and asymmetry, both seek to incorporate the real (personally expressive) and the analytic in ways that create a new kind of analytic relationship for the patient with real consequences for symbolization and growth. My participation in this crisis with Suzanne was improvised spontaneously, but I don't feel I left my role as analyst as we went through it. Our ritually based frame was temporarily breached, but my "inner frame" was present despite this alteration in our ritual. Moreover, as Hoffman (1998) argued, the tension I maintained between my humanness and analytic authority likely rendered the impact of my validation and prioritization of Suzanne's needs more potent as an antidote to the invalidating identifications with her internal objects.

Finally, in a different register still, this vignette could also be seen as a good illustration of certain principles from non-linear dynamic systems theory (Galatzer-Levy, 2002; Coburn, 2014). Suzanne's and my system had been evolving productively in certain ways, but had also been relatively stuck in others—especially Suzanne's deeper anxieties regarding my ultimate trustworthiness. The call from her former friend was a completely unpredictable intrusion into, and "perturbation" of, our system. It was also an example of a small event setting in motion a "cascade" of interactions leading ultimately to a dramatic reorganization of the system. Unlike the other frames of reference I have mentioned, this one could not have been influencing my thinking at the time since I had not yet incorporated complexity theory into my theoretical universe. But ironically, this fact offers a kind of backward support for one of the theory's therapeutic implications—the principle of autocatalysm (Coburn, 2014). In Coburn's words: "[In contrast to the traditional] notion that one person acting on or toward another is what effects change, [complexity theory] allows for the likelihood that the agent of change emerges as a product and property of the relational system itself" (2014, Kindle Edition, Introduction, "Attitudes": Attitude 4). This principle seems especially apt here in that, as I felt my way through the crisis with Suzanne, I was not *aware* of following any particular ideas about therapeutic action, including the ones reviewed above. The entire situation and the way Suzanne and I dealt with it were unique to our relationship and unprecedented in my experience. This is not to say that the other frames of reference weren't affecting me; I believe they were. Rather, it illustrates the complex relationship between complexity theory and psychoanalytic theories as they operate within and through the analyst's conscious and implicit subjectivity.

The preceding selective literature review is only a very partial conceptual rendering of the possible therapeutic factors operating in what took place between Suzanne and me. Pizer's (1998) seminal explication of "negotiation" as central to a relational analytic process, Benjamin's (2004) and Aron's (2006) various "intersubjective thirds," especially Benjamin's "moral third," Orange's (1995, 2008) stance of "emotional availability" growing out of her integration of the ethical philosophy of Emmanuel Levinas (1969), and Corpt's (2011) and Pizer's (2014) papers on clinical generosity, are only some of the other contemporary frames of reference that describe and help explain the transformative outcome of our crisis.

Conclusion

The upshot of this deconstruction of the therapeutic processes involved in Suzanne's and my crisis is that the creation (really, co-creation) of a needed analytic relationship in our contemporary psychoanalytic era is a complex matter. The proliferation and evolution of our psychoanalytic theories and frames of reference give us increasingly powerful lenses and reflective tools through which to observe and process the intersubjective happenings (and intrapsychic correlates) that constitute the analytic encounter. I believe this conceptual and procedural complexity represents an expansion of psychoanalytic wisdom, which deepens our understanding of what our patients need from us and frees us to act more creatively and humanly in response to those perceived needs.

Chapter 3

Fittedness and its vicissitudes

The word "fitted" might evoke images of physical objects being fitted to each other, like a puzzle piece being placed in its correct location, pie dough being molded to the contours of a pie pan, or a new garment being tailored to better conform to the owner's body. Such physical metaphors capture certain elements of psychoanalytic fittedness—for example, making interpretations in language the patient is likely to be able to understand and connect with, or adjusting the rhythms of silence and speech to what the analyst senses to be the patient's optimal processing rhythms. However, the full meaning of the concept, as Sander intended it and as I am using it here, is more complex and subtle. The analyst does not exactly exert conscious effort to take stock of the patient's current therapeutic needs and then consciously strive to meet them in some optimal way. Psychoanalytic interaction is too complex, moves far too quickly, and is too saturated with unconscious, implicit, and enactive elements for this kind of conscious, intentional, linear processing and reacting. Rather, fittedness is an *emergent property* of non-linear, dynamic processes that are constantly evolving within the patient-analyst dyad, situated within the more inclusive analytic field as it self-organizes and reorganizes over time. (See also Boston Change Process Study Group, 2010.)

But what does this really mean regarding the nature of the analyst's participation and the processes through which the patient's psychic reality (including the reality of his therapeutic needs) is apprehended, responded to, and transformed? In particular: (1) How do we think about the analyst's intentionality (especially the intention to achieve progressive fittedness), given the non-linear, unpredictable complexity of the analytic process and the trends in contemporary relational theory emphasizing more open, undirected attention, the capacity to dwell in uncertainty, and the unbidden arrival of new perception and understanding (Bion, 1970; D.B. Stern, 2013b)?

Moreover, (2) how do we think about the relationship between the intention to achieve progressive fittedness and all that is going on unconsciously, enactively, and spontaneously in the ongoing analytic exchange? In this chapter and the next, I approach these questions from a variety of angles.

The fundamental paradox

As a first step in unpacking the complexities of Sander's concept as applied in the analytic situation, it is useful to restate Principle #4 from the Introduction:

> Achieving progressive fittedness does not necessarily mean meeting the patient's needs on the terms that the patient is stating them or complying with some fantasized response the patient is enactively pulling for. Rather, it means *co-creating the therapeutic conditions* that best enable the patient to work and move toward her or his own mostly implicit therapeutic/developmental aims as these become actualized and articulated within the analytic setting over time.

If we were to apply Bion's (1959) terms for characterizing different kinds of group process to the analytic dyad, this principle offers a serviceable definition of the dyad as a "work group" as opposed to a "basic assumption group." A work group in Bion's scheme is a healthy-functioning group—i.e., one that is on task, able to face, cope with, and learn from reality, and thus move productively toward actualizing its aims or reasons for being. A basic assumption group, on the other hand, is one that has regressed into a less healthy mode of functioning, usually involving some form of implicit magical thinking: for example, a "dependency group." In a dependency group the members unconsciously adopt a *modus operandi* wherein the leader knows best, and the other members are ostensibly relying on the leader to guide them.[1]

As Principle #4 implies, for an analytic dyad to function as a work group a fundamental paradox must be recognized and reinvented uniquely and repeatedly in each case. The paradox could be, and has been, stated in different conceptual languages. Framing it in developmental terms, Sander (2008) conceived of it as the co-existence of two biological givens. The first is that each individual is a complex system that *tends toward self-organization and self-regulation*: "The agency to initiate action to self-regulate within the context of one's unique life support system must be the individual's own agency to initiate; [this is] the 'being distinct from' pole." The second is "the *capacity for microsecond synchrony and attunement with an 'other'* . . . the 'being together with' pole" (p. 167, emphasis added). "Both givens," Sander wrote, "are there from the beginning of life and provide the essential conditions for the experience of 'connection with' another and for the positive affects that are the basis of motivational systems underlying healthy relationships" (p. 167).

In the context of adult analytic therapy the dyadic system is set in motion and driven primarily by the first pole: *the patient's* struggles, motivations, initiatives, implicit aims, therapeutic needs, and unconscious communications. It has been an assumption of the psychoanalytic set-up from the beginning (Freud, 1913) that patients come with problems they are motivated to work on (or at least an illness they are motivated to remediate) and thus implicit aims toward which they are unconsciously, if ambivalently, motivated to strive. The free association method rested on this assumption—namely, that the patient would, if encouraged, spontaneously (mostly through unconscious choices) communicate what the analyst needed to know in order to understand and help with the core problems, assuming that the analyst was capable (through training) of receiving, processing and interpreting these communications. Freud also recognized the opposite current: Many of the patient's spontaneous communications reflect "resistances" to the truly free associations necessary to directly expose the warded off memories and problematic unconscious conflicts. However, in one of his many Zen-like insights, Freud (1912a) came to understand that the resistance itself, especially as expressed through the transference, was a necessary, expectable starting point, and, with skillful confrontation and interpretation, the *way into* the patient's core anxieties and conflicts.

This basic premise ("fundamental rule") creates a necessary space for the self-organizing pole in Sander's developmental paradox. But as Sander posits in development, and relational theorists from Winnicott (1965) and Bion (1962) to Ogden (1994) have similarly posited in adult treatment, this impetus to initiate, communicate, and direct always exists, *indeed, only comes into existence*, in an intersubjective surround defined by the necessary asymmetrical, primary relationship (infant-caregiver; patient-therapist), within which such communications are (at least potentially) received, recognized (attuned to), and responded to in needed ways.

It is only when seen through the lens of this fundamental paradox that the concept of progressive fittedness, and the necessary conditions of the psychoanalytic dyad as a work group, come into focus. Progressive fittedness evolves from the cumulative co-creation of intersubjective or field conditions that facilitate *the patient's* movement in the direction(s) of his own implicit developmental/reparative aims, recognizing that the nature and understanding of these implicit aims and needs are themselves to some degree shaped, if not generated, by the evolving intersubjective conditions. Ghent (1990) articulated this last feature of the paradox as follows:

> By "need" I am not implying that there is something like an inborn instinct for the integration of self. My view rather is that in normal development the most primitive functions and needs of an infant, when adequately responded to and interacted with by the environing others, give rise to ever more sophisticated and complex conative structures, which later we recognize as having the valence or motivational quality of need.
>
> (p. 112)

The need to make space for and respect the patient's initiative, has been recognized, at least implicitly, in the psychoanalytic operating assumption that it is the patient who must lead (with his associations as well as spontaneously arising behaviors and communications of all kinds), and the therapist who must follow the patient's lead and initiatives, gradually learning from these how best to respond and facilitate the patient's movement in the directions *he* is attempting to move.

The other side of the paradox is that, at the same time that the patient is leading and the analyst following, in another sense the analyst is leading and the patient is following. The analyst leads by bringing all of her analytic faculties and creativity to bear on the present moment of encounter, seeking to co-create through the total dialogue (verbal/implicit; conscious/unconscious) a place of meeting, a *communicative medium,* that the patient can use in the present moment to move forward (or inward) in ways she was not necessarily aware she even wanted or needed to move. This leading function does not rely on some imagined omniscience on the analyst's part; rather, only on the analyst trying to do her job of meeting the patient, using the tools at hand. However, as I emphasized in Chapters 1 and 2, the more tools the analyst has at hand the greater her potential for co-generating the "simple complexity" needed for successive approximations of fittedness.

This more complex understanding of fittedness makes it clear that the analyst's help cannot take the form of slavish tracking, attunement, or provision (where provision could refer to any form of therapeutic intervention, from interpretation to empathy to relational expressiveness, depending on the therapist's ideas about therapeutic action). Rather, the co-creation of fittedness relies on the analyst's relative freedom of thought and movement (Symington, 1983; Ehrenberg, 1992; Ogden, 1994; D.B. Stern, 2013c; S. Stern, 2009c, Chapter 6 in this book), her openness to the complexity and "feeling" of what is happening (to paraphrase Damasio, 1999), or what Havens (1989) evocatively called "loose holding," from which place both the patient's and the therapist's improvisational gestures emerge.

Intentional participation←→open, undirected attention

The preceding section describes certain aspects of the analytic frame—the intersubjective role relationship and field conditions necessary for the emergence of progressive fittedness. Assuming this basic relational structure, how do we think about the relational processes through which the analytic dyad moves fitfully toward progressively inclusive, and hence progressively fitted, relational integrations? If our implicit intention is to work toward increasingly facilitating understanding and relational conditions, how do we reconcile that intention with the non-linear, unpredictable, emergent complexity of the analytic process and the trends in contemporary relational theory emphasizing more open, undirected attention, the capacity to dwell in uncertainty and the unknown, and the unbidden arrival of new perception and understanding?

I would argue, first of all, that the idea that an analyst can approach the analytic process without intention is absurd. We all intend to help our patients, and, to slightly refocus what was said in the Introduction: Every psychoanalytic theory, every psychoanalytic book and paper ever written, has been created and published in large part to influence the quality of attention and intention with which analytic therapists approach analytic work. Even publications championing the unintentional and unbidden would not be written unless the authors were seeking to educate and influence the quality of the analyst's intentions.

To enter more fully into the paradoxes involved, consider one of the most radical and famous statements regarding the importance of the analyst's openness and non-directed attention: Bion's (1967, 1970) injunction to approach each session "without memory or desire." At a purely logical level, the injunction is at least paradoxical, if not self-contradictory, in that Bion is describing an *intention* to approach each session without any particular intention! (See also Chapter 6.) But beyond the logical paradox, Bion's injunction, which calls for a kind of attentional neutrality or emptiness, is also meant as a *positive* statement intended to evoke a certain kind of positive attitude in the analyst. Bion described it as a "positive discipline . . . a positive act of refraining from memory and desire" (1970, p. 31). Bion's statement is intended to encourage attentional receptivity and openness with an eye to that which is not yet known or is even unknowable. It also has the implication that by freeing herself as much as possible from both preconception and the registers of memory and sensory experience, the analyst brings into play *intuition* as a primary mode of apprehension—intuition, in Bion's view, being the necessary register for apprehending the psychic phenomena most relevant to psychoanalysis. The overall positive intention contained in Bion's dictum has a mystical quality: a uniquely psychoanalytic "faith" that, freed of memory and desire, the analyst will be in the best position to achieve "at-one-ment" with the total reality (the "O") of the session—a state of being from which new understanding (and thus useful intervention) has the best chance of "evolving."[2]

Translated into the language of fittedness, Bion is essentially saying that approaching the session with intentionally undirected, non-desiring attention is the best way to apprehend the psychic reality of the patient and the session and thereby ultimately generate understandings and interventions that *evolve from* and thus are *best fitted to* these psychic realities.

Another important element in Bion's recommended analytic attitude was what Keats (1817) had called "Negative Capability . . . that is, when a man is capable of being in uncertainties, mysteries, doubts, without any irritable reaching after fact or reason" (cited in Bion, 1970, p. 125). Influenced by Bion, Bollas (1987) spoke of states of confusion and uncertainty in the countertransference, which analysts must be able to "live in," sometimes for prolonged periods. And Ogden (e.g., 1994, 1997), also strongly influenced by Bion, demonstrates this capability in his narrative accounts of long periods of not knowing, accompanied by reveries whose meanings as transference-countertransference developments revealed themselves only in their own time and as a function of Ogden's radical openness (surrender) to them.

This principle of uncertainty also involves the patient, for it is the patient's responses (conscious and unconscious, immediate and delayed) to our interventions that are the truest tests of their fittedness. Gill (1994) emphasized the importance of tracking a patient's total behavior during the sessions following an interpretation to gauge its true effects. Similarly, Ferro (2005) and Peltz (2012), following Bion, write about the patient's "returned look" ("*après coup*")—the patient's total registration (conscious and unconscious) of a given interpretation—as the ultimate test of its fittedness and generativity.

My purpose in reviewing Bion's recommendations regarding the analyst's *intention* and *attention* is to help clarify a core paradox in the concept of fittedness as a guide for analytic apprehension and participation. The paradox is that, in the spirit of Bion, I believe we *should* approach each session with maximum openness and an orientation toward that which is not yet known, or, in D.B. Stern's (1990) words, an orientation that "courts surprise." And the reason we should do this is *so that* what emerges are understandings and forms of relational engagement that are progressively fitted to the patient's psychic reality and therapeutic needs.

Contouring and the dimension of time

Bion and Stern instruct us how to orient to the present, always complex and unpredictable, analytic moment. The idea of *progressive* fittedness, however, implies a temporal dimension to the achievement of fittedness, and with this temporal dimension the paradox deepens. The progressive achievement of fittedness requires that over time certain very fluid, always-morphing, understandings emerge, which take a certain "shape" and thus come to involve certain kinds of "memory" and intention implicit in how one speaks to and interacts with the patient. It is essential that the understandings that ground the intentions be *loosely held (softly assembled)*, and exist side-by-side with attentional openness, so that they are always open to modification, adaptation to the uniqueness of each analytic session and moment, and potential disconfirmation as therapeutic conditions and understanding change. To this end, Bion (1987) advised approaching every session as if it were the first session. At the same time, it *can be* equally important that certain understandings, and the relational positioning that accompanies them, be held with increasing *conviction* because that very conviction is what the patient needs from the analyst in order to gradually, incrementally, change longstanding patterns of thought, affect, and behavior.[3]

My work with Linda described in Chapter 1 is a case in point. During the first few years of treatment, amid the full unpredictable complexity of how our relationship and co-created understanding were fitfully evolving, I gradually developed a conviction that Linda would need to somehow make more of a commitment to the regularity of analytic sessions in order to achieve her most central aims for the analysis.[4] This conviction stood in apparent opposition to Linda's need for unfettered freedom and control when it came to regulating the continuity and depth (degree of dependency) of her felt connection to me. Thus it was essential that I be attuned to and respectful of this opposing need for control *even as* I was asserting my conviction about the minimal conditions necessary for the kind of analytic work she had signed up for. It was in this sense that my evolving conviction existed side-by-side with the intention to experience and understand Linda exactly as she was (with me in each session), with no agenda or "desire" for her to be different, and always with an eye to what I had not yet understood. The brief sample of our process that I included in my case description offers a window into how this paradoxical stance played out in our language and process (Chapter 1, p. 39).

This may also be an example of what Bion (1962) referred to as "binocular vision"—experiencing psychoanalytic phenomena from two or more points of reference (vertices) simultaneously—except here the points of reference were ostensibly contradictory or at least paradoxical. And, in this case what was binocular was not just my vision of Linda but my *ways of being with and speaking to her*, which emanated from that binocular vision. The term I would use to characterize this complexity and specificity of approach is ***contouring***—a process of evolving an understanding and relational engagement (specificity of recognition and connection) that is contoured to each patient's unique and always-evolving complexity as expressed within the intersubjective, analytic field. Contouring is essentially synonymous with fittedness except that, as both a noun *and* a verb, it captures the fluid multi-dimensionality (including the dimension of time) and the co-created *feeling of form-in-motion* involved in the process of achieving fittedness. One yield of such contouring is a progressive deepening in the patient's feeling of *being known* by the therapist at a visceral as well as cognitive level. This connects with Sander's (1995) operationalization of the idea of specificity in recognition as "knowing oneself as one is known."

Thelen (2005), applying a complexity theory perspective to both development and psychotherapy, wrote:

> The developing system is so highly non-linear that even small events may cascade to have large consequences . . . Because the future course is largely unknown, the web of past causality can hardly ever be really unentangled . . . And now the good news: The very same time-dependent complexity that gives us this circular causality also provides multiple ways to change . . . As a person's stable patterns are the product of many interrelated organic and experiential factors, any number of those factors may also be an entry to disrupt those patterns. The job of a skilled therapist is to detect where the system is open to change, to provide the appropriate new input to destabilize the old pattern, and to facilitate the person's seeking of new solutions.
>
> (pp. 279–280)

Thelen's characterization of the therapist's job in the face of each patient's complexity provides a link between Bion's and Stern's emphases on moment-to-moment, session-to-session, undirected openness and my focus in this section on the movement through time toward progressive fittedness. Since each patient's unique complexity defies any linear or fixed model of therapeutic action, it is only through the progressive fittedness (contouring) of the therapist's understanding and "implicit relational knowing" (D.N. Stern et al., 1998), as it gradually evolves from many moments of meeting (in Sander's original sense), that she can sense the "interrelated organic and experiential factors" (p. 280) which provide potential "entry points" for destabilizing the patient's system.

Intentional fittedness ← → experiential and expressive freedom

Bion's injunction to approach each session without memory or desire concerns, primarily, the analytic therapist's *attentional* orientation. In this section I focus on a second, related dialectical tension: that between the analyst's intention or aim of achieving progressive fittedness and her *experiential and expressive freedom*. The core ideas are more fully elaborated in Chapter 6—"The Dialectic of Empathy and Freedom"—but are here reframed within the fittedness sensibility emphasized throughout this book.

The aim of achieving progressive specificity of recognition and connection represents a particular kind of therapeutic intention—an intention to grasp our patients' current and evolving states, their past, present and feared traumas, and their implicit developmental aims and relational needs, and to respond in ways that are optimally fitted to all that we perceive in a given moment. This aim or intention has convergences with the self-psychologist's intention to work toward increasingly empathic attunements to a patient's complex subjective experience, and to intervene in ways that communicate, explicitly or implicitly, that empathic grasp. The concept of fittedness, however, is more inclusive than that of empathic understanding and communication in that our patients often need more than our empathic resonance. They may need all kinds of other things, some of which fall into theoretically established categories of analyst participation—interpretation, confrontation, authentic self-expression, certain kinds of guidance or instruction, or assistance with affect-regulation—but many of which are forms of participation that evolve uniquely within each dyad.

Another way to say this is that an analytic relationship is fundamentally a *lived experience*: Patient and analyst *live through things together* and, in a very circumscribed way, *create a life together*. It is this real lived experience that has the power to heal the toxic, deeply inscribed effects of the patient's early life and past traumas. Seen from this perspective, it becomes clear that empathy, attunement, and understanding are necessary but not sufficient principles for a fully alive analytic experience. The lived relationship between patient and analyst is densely complex and the analyst is always partaking of this relational complexity and generating complex interventions from within it. In order to do this in a way that truly moves in the direction of "four-dimensional" fittedness requires a paradoxical or dialectical framing of the intention to achieve progressive fittedness itself.

In Bion's (1970) way of thinking, the intention to move toward progressive fittedness constitutes a form of "desire"—i.e., a theoretical preconception that potentially interferes with the analyst's apprehension and processing of the total intersubjective, psychic reality of the session. I would add that it can also interfere with the freedom necessary to *act* on the basis of that apprehension and processing.

My solution to this problem (elaborated more fully in Chapter 6) is to position the intention to move toward progressive fittedness in dialectical tension with *two* principles of analytic freedom. The first is the one already discussed: the freedom implied in Bion's injunction to approach the session free of memory and desire. This is essentially a freedom of apprehension and processing. The second is the intention to respond to the patient—to *act* within the analytic field based on one's apprehension and processing—*without any preconceived aim or intention*, except the over-arching intention to further the analytic process. This latter principle of *experiential and expressive freedom* needs always to be present to some degree to enable us to "move with" the current process in complex, unpremeditated, intuitive ways; but it is essential for navigating in situations of impasse, confusion, turbulence, and enactment when we need to somehow feel our way through without yet having a conscious, or even implicit, grasp of what is happening and what is needed. The following clinical example, excerpted from my 2002 paper, "Identification, Repetition, and Psychological Growth," illustrates the dialectical tension I am getting at.

Tom

Tom, a man in his mid-30s, came for therapy and ultimately analysis, because he was significantly depressed with frequent suicidal ideation. There were also serious sexual concerns. He felt he had a small penis and thus felt inadequate to satisfy women sexually despite considerable evidence to the contrary. For example, his girlfriend of 5 years was very affirming in this regard.

The family scenario for Tom, growing up, was that he had been enlisted by his mother as an ally in her relentlessly hostile relationship with his father. He regarded his mother as an embattled saint, devoted to her children but victimized by his angry, emotionally immature, intellectually limited father. Thus he devoted himself to making his mother happy by trying to be the kind of person he sensed she wanted him to be—responsible and high-achieving—and by defending her against the father's verbal attacks by getting in the middle and verbally attacking him himself.

In treatment, Tom's initial ways of engaging with me were complex and contradictory. He was skeptical that therapy could have much to offer that he, an intelligent, Ivy League-educated, introspective person, could not figure out for himself. Yet, at the same time, he seemed genuinely grateful for, and excited by, the insights into his current paralysis that I offered during the first few months of treatment. There were sessions in which he seemed in touch with his depression, the problems in his life and his increasing reliance on our relationship as a source of insight and hope. Just as often, however, he would come in in a more ironically detached mood and regale me with reports of his many cultural activities and the insights *they* had inspired. I noticed that in his reports of these activities he focused on the author as much as the work, emphasizing the author's brilliance or wisdom or originality, and how the author's ideas had given him new and meaningful insight into some aspect of himself or the world.

During this early period I began to be aware of a subtle sense of evaluative detachment in Tom's attitude toward me. It was clear he was scrutinizing me in terms of the intellectual value I added to his life, and the jury was still out. I found myself trying to be particularly sharp and incisive, preconsciously working to engage him. When I said something that obviously struck him I felt relieved and gratified. But when whole sessions or strings of sessions went by without any new insights from me, I could sense his disappointment and withdrawal. This was the uncomfortable atmosphere I was "living in" with Tom for some months, feeling anxiously uncertain of how to navigate.

As the tension built around this I felt I needed to say something. Finally, during a session in which Tom could barely contain his disgust that I had liked the movie *Good Will Hunting*, which he had hated, I expressed my awareness of how disappointed he obviously was in me. He admitted that, although he thought I was probably doing the right thing by not giving too many interpretations, he was having questions about how smart I was. Having said this, he immediately wondered if I felt like strangling him! I reflected for a moment and said, "No, but I'm aware of feeling alone in our relationship." He said, "That makes me feel sad. I know I keep a critical distance from everyone, and the more intense a relationship, the more dissatisfied I am." With this opening, I went on to interpret that I thought there was an addictive quality to his pursuit of what I called "intellectual orgasms," and that when he did not get these from me he felt intensely frustrated and disappointed. Obviously struck by this, he admitted that at times he wished he could be in analysis with Sigmund Freud, imagining that with Freud there would be one brilliant insight after another.

In the sessions following this interaction there was a sense of Tom's being less critically detached. He revealed that he was having homosexual anxieties triggered by several homosexual dreams. In one he was sucking on a big penis. His own association was that it related to his father in some way. He said that he resonated to the idea that his intellectual strivings were connected to his sexuality and admitted that my interpretation had confirmed his own suspicion that there was something about his intellectual life that was not all healthy. He had always been afraid that he was not capable of his own original thoughts and that he secretly relied upon the thoughts of others whose intellects he respected in order to appear intelligent. I interpreted that his compliance and identification with his mother's expectation that he devote himself to her over his own development had left him out of touch with himself—his own feelings, needs, desires, perceptions, and beliefs. He did not know who he was, thus had no sound basis for guiding his own life. At the same time, her expectations that he be intellectually high-achieving, and that he protect her from his father, placed him in a position of having to act more mature, intelligent, and man-like than he felt, with no hope of receiving the positive experiences with his father that might have helped him in this regard.

This sequence of interpretations seemed to reach Tom in a new way. He said "I've always felt embattled, always had to show my big ideas, my big thought. It's exhausting. I always had to have an intellectual erection, yet I felt so inadequate sexually." In the following session he reported having had better sex with his girlfriend, during which he had not felt small. Several sessions later he reported having cried the night before "because I realized that ideas are less important than feelings." He also reported having told his girlfriend about a fantasy he had of crawling into my lap like a child (2002b, pp. 732–734).

Discussion

This vignette, which, in the original paper, was used to illustrate a different set of theoretical ideas, is here re-presented as an example of the dialectical interplay between the aim of achieving progressive specificity of recognition and connection and the freedom necessary to experience and respond to the patient from within the current, infinitely complex, mostly unconscious, transference-countertransference situation. What happened in this sequence of course reflects my idiomatic style of being and working and the unique intersubjective complexity of Tom's and my process early in our "analytic life" together. In hindsight, I can see clearly how

Tom's initial stance of evaluating my therapeutic value against impossibly high standards was unconsciously evoking my own early experience with my similarly critical-evaluative mother, undoubtedly contributing to my anxiety and pre-conscious efforts to prove myself to him, and impairing my capacity to think freely about how to be Tom's analyst during this period. One might say that, during this early, uncomfortable, months-long impasse, Tom and I were unconsciously "fitting together" mostly (though not entirely) in old, repetitive, enactive ways.

Things came to a head (as they needed to) with Tom's uncontrolled expression of disgust at my positive response to *Good Will Hunting*. My first reaction—reflecting how "obviously disappointed" Tom was in me—seems to me a subtly complex intervention. In one sense it was a relatively traditional and obvious mirroring of Tom's attitude and affect in that moment—a gesture toward empathic fittedness. At the same time there was a subtle act of freedom (Symington, 1983) in my willingness to take Tom and me into "the eye of the storm" that had been brewing between us.

By naming Tom's intense disappointment with me while hinting at, yet also containing, my own reactive affects, I implicitly invite Tom to fully "go there," as if to say: "OK, I'm ready to hear what you've been thinking about me—in fact, it's important for you to tell me." Tom hears this and does go there—trying to be tactful as he ruthlessly shares his real concern about my intelligence, then worries that I will feel like "strangling" him. Now we *are* in the eye of the storm, and in a kind of "now moment" (D.N. Stern et al., 1998)—an emergent, fateful moment in which what I do next matters a lot, and there are no roadmaps. In that moment I realize that what I'm feeling, pretty intensely, is not anger but a sense of being painfully alone and alienated from Tom, and I give myself the freedom to say it. This direct, spontaneous disclosure of my feelings in a vulnerable, non-retaliatory way has the effect of immediately transforming Tom's and my intersubjective field, enabling Tom, for the first time in the analysis, to risk sharing his own core feeling of sadness, and to reflect in an affectively real way on the distancing effect of his "constant attitude" (Reich, 1933) of critical detachment with significant others.

Now, suddenly in a more open, connected, "breathable" space with Tom, I feel freer to think and speak thoughts about his struggles that have been pre-consciously and unconsciously evolving in me over the preceding months. In language that feels fully alive to (my sense of) Tom's unconscious truth, I begin to interpret the addictive quality of his intellectual life, the link between his sexual and intellectual selves through the common experience of smallness and inadequacy in both domains, and the disabling oedipal scenario with his parents, in which he was still very much caught up. My explicit, edgy, highly personalized or contoured language has an apparently freeing effect as Tom joins me in elaborating the metaphor of his need for intellectual orgasms. Over the next few sessions, he is able, for the first time, to play with me and his own unconscious as he allows himself to explore and make connections regarding some of the core organizing principles (Stolorow & Atwood, 1992) through which he has been living and constricting his life. While I suspect that his dream of sucking a big penis has likely transference elements—perhaps reflecting his feeling homosexually seduced or fed by my "phallic" interpretation of his quest for intellectual orgasms—my intuition is not to pursue it in this context, but rather to allow his process as much space as possible for his own unconscious creative work. I do offer an extended genetic interpretation explaining his reliance on the wisdom of others as an understandable deficit, given all of the forces pulling him away from his own self-development up until this point in his life. While the interpretation has a didactic quality, it is also empathic to his unconscious experience, and he is able to make real use of it in recognizing the "embattled," "exhausting" nature of his struggle to stay afloat in the particular cross-currents of his real and internalized intersubjective world. Finally, he reaches a point of sufficient comfort with his own vulnerability with me to have and share the fantasy of crawling up into my lap like a trusting child in need of letting go and being soothed—a beginning movement, at least in fantasy, toward *surrender*, which Ghent (1990) believed lies at the heart of the psychoanalytic healing and self-healing process.

Stepping back from the interaction, I would say that giving myself the experiential and expressive freedom to share my countertransference feelings with Tom (feeling alone in our relationship) is what made possible, in a completely un-premeditated way, a whole new form of fittedness between us—my authentic relational response, which immediately called forth the same from Tom—thereby quickly deepening (in a generative and highly contoured metaphorical language) both our relational connection and shared dynamic understanding of major dimensions of his implicit experience of self-in-relation-to-others. As I have occasionally found in such exchanges, our transformative moment of meeting set in motion what dynamic systems theorists (e.g., Goldstein, 2007) call an "avalanche" or "cascade" of rapidly and progressively deepening understandings, with accompanying shifts in Tom's emotional insight, self-experience, and experience of me, leaving our "dynamic system" in a very different place than when we first entered "the eye of the storm."

* * *

The dialectical/paradoxical tension between the therapeutic intention to work toward progressive fittedness (specificity of recognition and connection) and the freedom to experience and respond to the present intersubjective, analytic moment without any particular intention is one of the conceptual "navels" of this book, with implications that radiate outward through many of the chapter themes and clinical examples. It is a dialectical tension that has its origins in Freud's (1912b) recognition that the analytic set-up ideally enables the analyst to process the patient's associations with enough unconscious freedom to arrive at understandings and interpretations that are increasingly fitted to the patient's complex psychic reality.

As will be discussed at greater length in Chapters 5 and 6, both Winnicott (1949, 1969) and Bion (1962, 1967, 1970) expanded and deepened Freud's original understanding. Each, in different but paradigmatically overlapping ways, recognized the importance of the analyst's freedom (conscious and unconscious), not only for purposes of cognitively processing the patient's material but also in order to provide certain essential developmental/relational functions such as (1) emotional containment (Bion, 1962), (2) survival of patients' aggressive/projective destructiveness (Winnicott, 1969), and (3) achieving a transformative "at-one-ment" with the psychic/intersubjective reality of the patient and the session (Bion, 1967, 1970). My "now moment" with Tom, in which I first invited the full force of his negative judgment, then shared my feeling of aloneness with him, could be understood as embodying all of these functions. In the same moment: (1) I was unconsciously processing, metabolizing, and returning to him (and myself) a frightening and previously uncontained dimension of his (our) affective experience; (2) I survived his critical destructiveness by sharing my emotional experience with him in a non-retaliatory way; and (3) I allowed myself to be "at one" with, or to fully enter, the immediate intersubjective reality of what was happening, thereby bringing Tom into a similar at-one-ment with his own emotional reality, and freeing both of our minds to penetrate more deeply into the nature of Tom's disabling experience of self-in-relation-to others.

The understanding of this same fundamental dialectic was further expanded, beginning in the 1980s, with the early relational contributions of Bollas (1987), Mitchell (1988), Ehrenberg (1992), Benjamin (1990), Hoffman (1992, 1994), Davies (1994), Ogden (1994), Aron (1996), Pizer (1998) and others in their collective recognition and elaboration of the therapeutic potential of the analyst's participatory, expressive freedom. From a fittedness perspective, each of these authors, in different ways, recognized and showed how the analyst's un-premeditated authentic responsiveness to the patient, especially in the most difficult, anxiety-producing situations and impasses, could, when held in tension with the analyst's reflective discipline, open up and transform the analytic process from repetitive, constricting forms of fittedness to new, freeing, growth-supporting integrations.

Notes

1 Bion identified other kinds of basic assumption groups as well, and we now might say that any kind of seriously challenging enactment constitutes movement of the dyad toward some form of basic assumption group. The focus in this section is on using Bion's concepts to flesh out my ideas about fittedness in the analytic situation. The points I make about the dyad as a dependency group could easily be generalized to all forms of basic assumption group dynamics. Like Ogden (2009), I view the relationship between basic assumption and work group dynamics as dialectical. That is, just as we cannot avoid enactments, we cannot avoid gravitating toward basic assumption group dynamics with our patients; the question is how we are able to process and learn from these modes of engagement and continually transform them into increasingly enriched and complex forms of work-group engagement.

2 I understand this analytic state as similar in certain respects to Ghent's (1990) concept of "surrender," but held as an *a priori* attitude or mental state rather than a case-specific *development*. Integrating Bion and Ghent, it would seem that the analyst's modeling the kind of contained surrender Bion advocated can be a necessary precondition for the patient's more contingent surrender as the process unfolds and deepens. See also Eigen (1981) for an extended meditation on the concept of "faith" in Winnicott, Lacan, and Bion.

3 Hoffman (1998) characterized this paradox as a dialectical tension and oscillation between *uncertainty* and *conviction.*

4 In taking a stance of this kind I was consciously assuming the role of "doctor," asserting, in effect, that, "if you (Linda) want this 'medicine' to work, you need to take it at the 'recommended dose.'" Relational analysts have, for many good reasons, grown increasingly uncomfortable with adopting such an authoritative stance (e.g., Mitchell, 1997, Chapter 2)—one that is all too reminiscent of the classical analytic attitude in its most doctrinaire, medicalized form. Yet, too thoroughgoing a repudiation of this role can work to the detriment of our patients, some of whom, at times, need us to assume responsibility for taking a strong position on their behalf. (See also Chapter 7 on the "Conundrum of Self Care".) This is a complicated area—one that bears closer attention. My own approach to it, illustrated in my work with Linda, is to hold such a stance dialectically (in tension with a more here-and-now, accepting, emancipatory attitude), and to be constantly mindful of the distinction between firmness or assertiveness and a more malignant need (often unconscious) to control the patient.

Chapter 4

The tendency toward fittedness and the forward edge of the relational unconscious

In Chapter 1 I raised the intriguing question of whether the spontaneous, almost magical, coordination we "observed" between the father and infant daughter in Sander's video clip has a counterpart in adult analytic dyads—that is, a *tendency toward fittedness* that is a property of the dyad as a similarly asymmetrical, developmentally purposed (although far more complex) dynamic system. If so, it would suggest that there is a forward tending dimension, not only of the patient's individual unconscious (Weiss, Sampson, et al., 1986; Newman, 1988; Bollas, 1989; S. Stern, 1994; Tolpin, 2002), but of the so-called "relational unconscious" (Lyons-Ruth, 1999; Gerson, 2004; Bromberg, 2011; Aron & Atlas, 2015) as well. The problem in addressing this question directly and discursively is the elusiveness of the phenomenon: If you try to look at it too directly, you won't see it; it can only be inferred from processes that occur "when you're not looking." To cope with this epistemological conundrum I will first present two clinical examples, then use those examples as a way into articulating my understanding of the principles involved. The first case focuses on the tendency toward fittedness in the initial meeting with a patient. The second follows a case in which fittedness emerges unpredictably in different forms over time.

The tendency toward fittedness in the first session

Beginning in the first session, patient and therapist are engaged in a complex process of feeling each other out: the patient trying to get a sense of whether this person can somehow help her, in a meaningful, effective way, work on problems in living she knows she has but, for the most part, can't really "see" and doesn't understand; and the therapist, using all of his faculties while listening (experiencing) in as relaxed and open a way as possible, trying to get a sense of who this unique person, with her unique life struggles, is (specificity of recognition), and of how to connect with her, mostly implicitly, though the exchange of words are central to this implicit sensing process (specificity of connection). This characterization, though structurally correct, doesn't fully capture the complexity of all the processes going on as a particular dyad begins to engage. If we think of what the observational methods used in contemporary infancy research can now show of the micro processes going on second-to-second between a mother and baby (e.g., Beebe & Lachmann, 2014), a similar kind of observational method applied to initial therapy sessions would no doubt reveal a comparable degree of intricacy and complexity in the new-patient-therapist interaction; and that doesn't take into account the added, unobservable, complexity of what each party is *thinking* from moment to moment as they interact. This complexity of intersubjective interaction going on, mostly out of awareness and in highly concentrated form in the first session, represents the beginning of a process of seeking, and moving toward, progressive fittedness, sensing with unusually heightened acuity (involving all of the senses and mental processing systems—cognitive and implicit) the potential pathways toward connection and useful communication as well as the potential obstacles and perceived risks to such integrations.

Winnicott (1971b), writing about first sessions with child patients, described his "squiggle" technique as "one way of getting into contact with a child . . . and of making the case come alive" (p. 3). I, as I'm sure many analytic therapists, think of first sessions with adults as a complex "squiggle game" between the total subjectivities of patient and analyst, both employing all forms of communication (verbal, affective, implicit, bodily, etc.) in an exchange that aims implicitly toward a first experience of fittedness—a preliminary experience on the part of the patient of "knowing oneself as one is known" (Sander, 1995). Winnicott regarded first sessions with children as "special occasions that have a quality that has made me use the word sacred" (p. 4). Sander (2008) conveys a similar feeling of awe and mystery as he describes the father-daughter interaction caught on video, which I quoted in Chapter 1. I regard first sessions with adults as similarly portentous, a literal moment of meeting, the hope for which is that the patient will leave feeling met in a new and promising way. I believe that underwriting this shared aim is a tendency toward fittedness operating "through" both parties as the system begins to form. Winnicott

(1971b) noted, in his review of the analytic competencies needed in order to facilitate such a mutual experience, that "one must have in one's bones a theory of emotional development of the child and of the relationship of the child to the environmental factors" (p. 3). As the example below attests, I am in full agreement with him.

By their nature, many first sessions might appear to an outside observer as if the patient is doing the majority of talking while the therapist mostly listens, passively and attentively, asking occasional questions. What all analytic therapists know to be the case, however, is that, as our patients communicate their stories, our minds—that is, all of our analytic faculties—are processing as much intersubjective data as possible and developing initial impressions and thoughts as part of a spontaneous "reaching for" fittedness in a myriad of different ways, including beginning to "grow the receptors and processors" we will need to develop to be able to meet a new patient in the "area" they are psychically inhabiting when they first arrive in our office. Moreover, my sense is that, even though I may not be giving much explicit verbal feedback, if my evolving thoughts, impressions, and feelings are, in fact, increasingly fitted to the patient's experience and struggles, the patient will somehow sense this attunement, and it will animate her narrative, sponsoring an implicit, bi-directional movement toward fittedness in an atmosphere of tentatively increasing promise and hope. In the example that follows I will indicate, using brackets, some of my silent thoughts and reactions.

Celeste

An attractive, put-together, articulate, and obviously very competent woman in her late 30s, Celeste's first statement of her problem was that she needed to "turn down my emotions" and that, especially with her sister, she had been "trying to feel less." She made these statements with obvious anxiety and urgency, clearly believing that however she had been expressing herself emotionally was destructive and wrong. [My first unspoken reaction (given that Celeste clearly did not have Borderline Personality Disorder) was that, whatever her problem was, this was not it. Not only do I believe it is impossible to "feel less" than one actually feels, I assume that this kind of thinking about oneself usually reflects some kind of "pathological accommodation" (Brandchaft, et al., 2010) to the requirements of one or more significant others.]

Her tone and facial expression changed somewhat as she next began to talk about her husband of 10 years, Tim. Showing an odd combination of facial strain and genuine warmth and pride, she described theirs as an "amazing partnership." The problem was that Tim "wants more sex" and "I don't feel it; I don't feel as interested." And she was very worried that this disparity would cause Tim to look elsewhere. She then brightened and said, "We have a great family, though," and "we're in business together!" Then the strain returned as she said that she was increasingly concerned about their "compatibility." Tim is "interested in adventurous sex—he likes to be dominated. I'm uncomfortable with that role." Shifting again, now with a tone of tentative agency, Celeste said Tim's "self-esteem is closely connected to what others think of him. I don't want to be responsible for his self-esteem." Shifting again to a tone of even stronger, more confident agency, she said: "I feel like I'm not getting enough attention from him. I feel like he's cheating, but not really."

She then explained that, although they were co-owners of their successful shared company, it was really his creation and reflected his interests and talents. In the last year he had unilaterally decided to start a new project that was consuming all of his time, leaving Celeste mostly on her own to manage the parent company—a role for which she did not feel fully competent. She needed his help with certain things, and felt that Tim, while giving lip service to his availability, had been seriously neglecting her, causing her to feel hurt, unrecognized, overwhelmed, and jealous, but also humiliated as if she *should* be able to do the things he expected from her. Then, herself making an unconscious link between the sex and work issues, she said: "I ask for verbal 'foreplay,' but that doesn't fit with his needs." She said: "We make love once a week, maybe," clearly feeling unhappy with this frequency.

[As Celeste has gone through this initial part of her story, essentially uninterrupted by me, I am experiencing an odd combination of inchoate feelings and senses. I sense that the dynamics with her husband are linked to those with her sister (and, I am assuming, her family of origin), but seem more complex. She clearly loves her husband, but feels caught somewhere in between accommodating his stated and implicit needs and trying to speak up for her own. She does some of the latter, reflecting some sense of self and agency, but she and Tim are in a kind of stand-off in which there is a large measure of her feeling it is a failing on her part that she isn't the way he wants her to be, and that she better work harder to get with the program or he might "cheat" on her and she could lose him. That is, his narcissistic needs are assumed to be a given; so she faces the impossible dilemma of either unhappily acceding to them or asserting her needs more forcefully at the risk of losing him. Hearing all this, I feel I understand these kinds of dynamics and can probably help her with them. But I'm also feeling somehow unmoved and not fully engaged. Something about the combination of needing to present herself as competent, conscientious, and up-beat while clearly battling a sense of strain, resentment, and fear that she might lose it all, has a subtly repellent effect on me that doesn't fit with her objectively appealing qualities. I feel uneasy.]

As if on cue, Celeste said, "Sometimes I'm afraid to open up. I'm outwardly open and friendly but inwardly guarded." [I immediately feel less uneasy and more engaged.] "This thing with my sister has torn our family apart." She then told the story of her family history—the parts she felt were relevant to her current struggles. Her parents immigrated to this country as young adults. Her older sister, and only sibling, has had serious mental problems—"anxiety, depression, maybe bi-polar"—and, from an early age, became her mother's "lifelong project." They are "co-dependent." The parents are still together but sleep in separate bedrooms. The father, a successful engineer, was and still is gone most of the time. He was a "great dad, but not a great husband." The mother, in Celeste's analysis, felt emotionally unfulfilled and isolated in a strange culture; hence the enmeshment with the sister. [Here, I note silently Celeste's generous justification for her mother's overly close relationship with the sister.]

I wondered out loud: "If your father was gone so much, how could he have been a great dad?" It didn't take much reflection for Celeste to say that, in fact, she felt mostly neglected by him, but had positive memories of his helping her with homework: Science had been hard for her and he was brilliant in that area. On closer look, she admitted that the help was very occasional, much less than she needed or would have wanted. When it happened she would be thrilled to have his attention and help, but he typically just told her what to do, or did it himself, rather than actually working with her to help her learn. Here I saw, and noted out loud, a connection between what she felt with her father and is now feeling with her husband at work. The connection had never occurred to her because of the idealization of her father—an idealization I assumed to have been necessary, given the more conflictual and infuriating relationship with her mother.

The sister was described as pretty much all take and no give. When she divorced her husband, Celeste felt more allied with the ex-husband. But the mother is very controlling when it comes to the sister, and uses guilt to pressure Celeste to be more sympathetic and supportive with her. [It is not hard to pick up Celeste's longstanding resentment of both her mother and sister. While she has no problem admitting her anger (more like hatred) toward her sister, she seems to need to view her relationship with her mother as positively as possible.] She admitted she has "conflicting feelings" toward her mother and feels "sad for her that she lost me." [I think: That last comment feels fishy. Who's taking care of whom in that relationship?] She described ups and downs with her mother since she became an adult. She wants to feel closer to her, and says things have improved in recent years. But there is a pattern of trying hard to be positive (as her mother implicitly requires), but then losing it in occasional outbreaks of rage, which cause things to deteriorate, sometimes for long periods of time. [Here, I remember how she began the session: "I need to turn down my emotions." I am thinking that unconsciously she still needs and longs for her mother to be a real mother to her; she tries to find evidence that this is the case and tries hard to be the person her mother seems to need her to be. But over and over the mother shows her true colors—namely that her (the mother's) needs almost always take precedence, and her main interest in Celeste is using her (the "strong" sister) to help her, the mother, help the "sick" sister in one way or another. She gives lip service to wanting to be there for Celeste but only rarely comes through for her in a real way. Celeste feels hurt and enraged about this, but then turns this into guilt at being the unpleasant person her mother accuses her of being.

The end of the session is approaching, and I can sense Celeste looking to me for something that will help her with her urgent fears and anxieties—her sense that she needs to get a hold of herself quickly and find a way to make it work with Tim. Why aren't I feeling more emotionally engaged, more moved by Celeste's painful history and current struggles, even as I know I want to work with her and believe I can help? I see a person working so hard all the time to make things work: with Tim, with her mother, with her job; trying to be herself (express her feelings and needs) with her most significant others, but always seeming to run up against the immovable narcissistic needs of the other and having little success commanding more of a true dialogue that yields something for her as well as the other. I'm aware that I could say something like this to Celeste, but really it would only amount to reflecting back to her what she has already told me. In any case, I am more focused on my disquieting feelings, and at that point have two virtually simultaneous revelations. The first is the painful recognition that Celeste's story is not unlike my own. I, too, feel like I have often, throughout my life, wanted more from others than they have been able or willing to give. The second is the realization that what I am feeling with Celeste seems to be a version of the very problem she has been telling me about: She has been working hard to get something she needs from me, but somehow acting in a way that makes me feel not fully connected and not fully inclined to give it to her. Then I think of all she has told me, and in every instance I see her being isolated in the midst of a successful life with ostensibly "normal" family relationships. And I think: Whatever happened to her as a child she now must be unconsciously recreating in her adult relationships. Finally, I know what I want to say.]

"As I've been sitting with you, listening, I'm aware of feeling like we're not quite connecting, even though I'm very much here with you and feel I do connect with your struggles. As I think about everything you have told me, I see you alone in every scene, even in the midst of a full, in many ways satisfying, life and even with the people you love the most. It makes me think you must be doing something unconsciously that perpetuates that state of aloneness." Hearing this, Celeste began quietly crying, and was basically speechless for the duration of the session. We both sensed that what I had said was true. And I felt I had intuited a way to "meet" her in a "place" she would not even have said she was occupying when the session began. This understanding became a central organizer for the twice-a-week treatment that followed, during which she was able to come to better terms with, and begin to grieve, what she had never really gotten from her parents, and to more fully claim her sense of agency in a way that enabled her to renegotiate and deepen her relationship with Tim and create a more viable role for herself at work.

Discussion

Even though, at the outset of this first session, Celeste could not have identified her core feelings of aloneness, I believe that at the *forward edge of her unconscious*, as it interacted with mine over the course of the session, she was reaching for needed recognition of the painful emotions that lay just under the surface of her story, with its multiple iterations of the same basic problem. At the same time, not only my conscious processing of her self-presentation, but my unconscious response to her unconscious warded off pain and need for recognition, was moving, if fitfully, toward an unconscious collaboration. In retrospect, I can see this unconscious interaction reflected in one of the few things I actually said: "If your father was gone so much, how could he have been a great dad?" This was not a planned question, and the affect it contained was spontaneous. I see it now as the kind of pointed question Sullivan (1954) might have asked: "kicking the props out from under" the incongruity in her narrative so as to get a "clearer picture" of the actual interpersonal situation, while, at the same time, emboldening the patient to feel "less than wonderful" about the father's actual participation in her life.[1] The deeper meaning for Celeste was the implied recognition of the painful feelings I was hearing between the lines of her account—a spontaneous gesture on my part toward recognition and fittedness. But I don't believe it was this one poignant question that connected Celeste's and my unconsciouses; it was all that was going on in the implicit exchange—not just in our (potentially) observable non-verbal *behavior*, but in all that was going on intersubjectively, including our conscious and unconscious mentation.

This example is also interesting and illustrative because there was a simultaneous unconscious enactment going on throughout most of the session. Side by side with my unconscious movement toward understanding, collaboration, and fittedness, I felt an inexplicable, disturbing lack of full, sympathetic engagement. In hindsight, clearly part of this had to do with my own history and unconscious identification with Celeste's particular kind of pain in relation to significant others, and part had to do with something she was unconsciously recreating in all of her important relationships. I believe that because my *primary* orientation was and is toward the question, "What does the patient need from me?" rather than "What's going on around here?" I was able to use the second question in service to the first. Thus my insight into both Celeste and myself in the last minutes of the session emerged from my struggle with my resistance to giving her what she seemed to need, and from my assumption that this struggle must carry information about what she needed from me at a deeper level. It was in this moment of anxious disequilibrium and uncertainty, a moment at "the edge of chaos" (Galatzer-Levy, 2002; Coburn, 2014; Marks-Tarlow, 2011), that my more deeply fitted interpretation spontaneously emerged.

The emergence of fittedness over time

Sam

Sam, a successful entrepreneur whose mother had died of cancer when he was 3, and whose financially successful, sociopathic father had remarried three times during his childhood, has been seeing me for about a year. He seems very happy to be coming to my office twice a week and has no trouble talking about his life, filling our hours with monologue—mostly stories of daily interactions with others that demonstrate both his business prowess and unusual generosity—which he seems to trust I will somehow, ultimately, be able to make use of. Indeed, despite a nagging sense of directionlessness on my part, Sam clearly has felt a deepening connection with me. He considers me one of the most trusted people in his life and obviously feels very warmly toward me. Some months into the analysis he asked if he could hug me at the conclusion of some sessions if he felt like it. I would ordinarily be quite uncomfortable with doing that, and have in the past actually refused certain patients' similar requests. But I found myself willing to try it with Sam. He now hugs me on his way out of every session, and I have come to experience it as a comfortable, meaningful ritual in our relationship.

For the most part I have allowed the process to evolve in a way Grossmark (2012a) might approvingly characterize as going with "the flow of enactive engagement," and Galatzer-Levy (2009) might similarly appreciate as the emergence of a pattern of "coupled oscillators."[2] I look forward to Sam's sessions, and enjoy listening to the rolling narrative of his daily exploits. We have evolved a particular kind of light-hearted, humor-infused, repartee that feels enlivening and affectionate in an analytically contained way. I think of Galatzer-Levy's paper and can feel temporarily reassured: Sam and I have a kind of synchrony together (Sander, 2002), a "rhythmic third" (Benjamin, 2002), which undoubtedly is connecting us and constitutes a new, grounding relational experience for Sam. Within this frame I can think: Maybe this is enough, and I shouldn't worry about it. Yet there is something in the quality of our sessions that troubles me. Although Sam free associates in a sense, with no difficulty, I often feel it is circular and somehow dissociated, but from . . . what? His core self? His suppressed/repressed affects? What's missing? Something. I sit in the sessions knowing I could let him go on for the entire time without any sense of traction or deepening. It is a coupled oscillator but one that seems to be going nowhere. If anything different is going to "happen" I will be the one who has to make it happen, or so it seems. In a sense, perhaps, this is always true with all of our patients. If they could make something happen on their own, they wouldn't need us. But with Sam, I feel that in simply listening to him, and joining him in what feels like a dialogical high, I am somehow remiss. Thus, there is always the question of what to do about it, if anything. Do I just let him go? Do I try to somehow redirect him toward . . . toward what? Do I talk about this conundrum and wonder out loud what is going on? What can he be trusted to do? What is my job?

Then one day, toward the end of a typically unsettling session, I had the thought: He speaks but I can't locate the *author* of his speech? It's as if speech happens, but without an inner speaker. Or if there is an inner speaker, "he" is not speaking primarily through the content of his words but through their impact as a kind of enactment or emotional communication. I told Sam that *he tells me stories, but I can't tell who the author is, or what his purpose is in telling me*. His reaction seemed to be somewhere in between being taken aback and lighting up. But we didn't have time to discuss it.

He began the next session making a joke indicating that what he had taken from the last session was that I was against "storytelling." I wondered if he felt wounded by my comment about authorship, as if I were criticizing him for not doing analysis right. I tried to clarify that this was not the case: I sensed behind *all* of his speech, not only his story telling, a kind of directionlessness. He said he operated with the understanding that I would learn something from his storytelling that would be useful. I said that demonstrated my point: He didn't sense a direction within himself. He spoke of wanting, at some level he knew wasn't realistic, a guru who would point him toward truth and direct him about how to live. He denied that I was that person, and claimed he wouldn't want me to be: He would just reject it. I said the wish for a guru also suggested he feels he doesn't have a clue and needs outside direction. Yes, he agreed, he was starting to see that, while he was the master of outside reality in certain ways, he felt cut off from his own reality—had no internal anchors. We revisited a comment of his wife, Carla, he had told me about previously: that he lives in an isolation tank, as in the 1980s film, *Altered States*. I said I felt that with him too. It's not just that he's cut off from inner reality, but also from others. It's the same basic barrier.

His acknowledgment that he was cut off from his internal reality and didn't know how to navigate felt like the truest, most real thing he had ever said to me, and I told him so. He then brought up that maybe both of us were swimming around in such complexity that we would just flounder together. I interpreted this as his worry that I wouldn't be able to help him, just as no one ever had. He agreed, but also reemphasized his trust and faith in me. He became almost tearful at this point, in obvious gratitude. He wondered what could help us. His dreams, he wondered? Yes, I answered. He got out a little notebook in which he had apparently jotted down some dreams—He'd been dreaming heavily, he said. As background to telling me about one of his dreams (which we never got to), he reported about his irritation with Carla in Washington D.C. on a recent vacation with their kids. On a number of occasions she had "rattled on" in complaint about being stuck in long lines waiting for things. This irritated him enormously. He felt like he was dealing with another child rather than a partner. He had gotten very critical and superior with her around this. I said his irritation tells us about him too. He has an allergy to her childlike states because they remind him of his traumatized inner child. He said, "You mean the 3-year-old (the age when his mother died)?" "Yes!" I exclaimed. He said, "But I think I started to become thoughtful and self-controlled in the way I am today very early." Yes, I agreed, but not before 3. He reflected and said he remembered reflecting on certain issues (in an extremely precocious way) when he was 4. Yes, I agreed, he's been taking care of himself since then: "*There's the 3-year-old and the 4-year-old*." At this, he became tearful again, and indicated that he was having a lot of feeling. The session ended and on the way out he hugged me more tightly, and in a more prolonged way, than ever before. I felt moved, and very close to him.

In the following session Sam revealed that he had dreamt about me for the first time. All he remembered was that I was with him and his family, as if I were virtually a family member. When I asked for his associations, he said it was about feeling safe with me. In this and the subsequent session I was aware of feeling more connected with him. He was more spontaneously reflective about his feelings, not just telling me stories but trying to locate himself in or behind them.

In short, what had emerged in three sessions of improvisational dialogue was a new purchase on an elusive but profound dislocation in Sam's experience of life. While he organizes his life so that he is always taking care of others, there is an inner 3-year-old who is still floundering, reeling from a totally unprocessed trauma, and unconsciously waiting for someone somehow to provide the help, direction, and care he is just beginning to recognize he needs.

* * *

Now, several years after the sessions I just described, I see that this extended interchange marked a turning point in our shared understanding, and a move toward progressive fittedness at a more complex level. The overall nature and tone of our sessions has not changed in a dramatic way. But Sam and I now both understand that his positive, lighthearted, hyper-competent narrative is the voice of what he now calls his "exoskeleton"—the precocious child-now-adult who needed to find a way to survive in the midst of trauma and chaos. He did so by, for the most part, dissociating his needs and pain, adopting a set of values and ethics opposite to his father's, and learning somehow to self-administer a kind of endorphin high through his determined positive attitude, success drive, and business acumen. Understanding this, I now hear moments in his narrative that glancingly refer to emotional pain he experiences in disappointing, hurtful, or frightening interactions with Carla and his children, or in his work life. His relationship with Carla has become increasingly painful and disappointing in ways that suggest she has become the stand-in for the mother who "abandoned" him at age 3, and the subsequent stepmothers, all of whom also ultimately abandoned him. These chinks in the exoskeleton are windows into his inner turbulence which is still so frightening to him that when we touch on it he immediately dissociates into a hypnoid state bordering on sleep. We joke about his avoidance, but he can acknowledge his fear that if he lets himself "go there" he will break down and cease to be able to function at the high level he unwaveringly sustains. We also joke about the question of who wants him to go into these painful feelings—me or him! He says he needs me to guide him, which in a way I do. But I know he will have to be the one to allow himself to "feel his feelings." I lead by marking the moments when he touches on feelings, but then allow him to go wherever he chooses, which is mostly, still, very quickly into a dissociated place. That is the current state of our fit.

Discussion

My treatment of Sam puts the concept of fittedness through its paces. We fell easily into a comfortable form of fittedness—a coupled oscillator

(Galatzer-Levy, 2009)—which clearly had therapeutic elements. At the implicit level, I believe it felt to both of us that our way of being together was important to Sam as the one place in the world where the needed asymmetry was firmly intact. As was revealed in my clinical narrative, Sam had to become very prematurely responsible for himself. Not mentioned was the fact that he also had to become responsible, at least in his own mind, for the significant adults in his life. After his mother died, Sam became aware very early that his father was ruthlessly and recklessly self-focused, impulse-ridden, prone to losing control of his anger, and unreliable as a parent cognizant of his children's feelings and needs. Sam implicitly realized he would need to be the one to "watch out for" his father rather than the other way around. Yet, he was unquestioningly "devoted" to his father as "the only person who stood between me and oblivion." There were similar role reversals in his relationships with several of his stepmothers, who came to use Sam as a confidante regarding his father. This role relationship carried into his adult life, expanding to include his whole relational world—a world in which he was, to use his word, the "capacitor": always judiciously building his resources in order to take care of himself, those he loves, and the many people from the community and beyond who come to him for advice or help of one kind or another.

Thus, I believe now, and sensed all along, that there were important therapeutic aspects to this way of "fitting together" that evolved between us—a forward edge dimension. There was a holding quality to the rhythms of our being-together, and to the fact that therapy was the one place where Sam could come, let down, and know that he had an appreciative, unconditionally receptive audience, not unlike the function good-enough parents serve for their children who are still at the age when they want to tell their parent(s) everything that happened at school or on some adventure.

At the same time, this way of fitting together felt disquietingly circular and undirected—an example of what D.B. Stern (2010) calls "chafing." Not wanting to disqualify either of these senses, but not seeing how to reconcile them, fittedness then took the form of living with and holding this uncertainty and confusion without too much "irritable reaching after fact or reason" (Keats, 1817, cited in Bion, 1970, p. 125). I would share my concern with Sam, but he viewed this as my problem; he was content to proceed and leave it to my analytic machinations to figure it all out. Then somehow, from this prolonged state of unsettling ambiguity and worry, the thought that I could sense "no author" behind Sam's stories emerged unbidden (Galatzer-Levy, 2002; D.B. Stern, 2013c). This emergent metaphor felt immediately relieving because I finally had language that fit my complex experience with Sam. Sharing my revelation with him seemed to crack open the months-long stalemate and set in motion a "cascade" of relational events.

The improvisational, much more fast-paced, dialogue that ensued was unlike any that had occurred previously, both of us speaking in slightly different voices with each other. It would be hard to say "what" exactly was guiding that dialogue, especially the "selected facts" (Bion, 1962) I chose to focus on: Sam's reaction to Carla complaining as she waited in long lines; the sudden realization that Sam's irritability with her must be connected to his own child-self in some way; and the way Sam and I established exactly when his precocious, exoskeletal self began to form and why. These improvisational exchanges were, to use the Boston Change Process Study Group's (2008) term, "sloppy." The thinking was inexact and the exchange moved quickly like an unguided, or rather semi-guided, missile, headed we knew not where as our newly enlivened dialogue proceeded. Yet, this improvisational dialogue generated one opening after another—in memory, dreams, understanding, and affect—and a deepening connection that was emerging simultaneously. By the end we were in a very new place, and the disquieting sense of directionlessness finally had started to come into focus in a useable way. It had become clear that Sam's child-self, which had been extremely well camouflaged by his hyper-competent adult self, was operating at the level of a traumatized (and probably regressed) 2 or 3-year-old, in need of a mother to perceive and meet very early needs for structure, regulation, guidance and holding he could hardly have known he had. These insights left me with new clarity about what Sam needed from me based on a new grasp of his psychological organization and its developmental origins.

Thus, in sum, although we can't exactly see the forward-edge workings of the relational unconscious, I believe we can sense it operating—pulling Sam and me forward through our efforts to "join our directionalities" in the service of Sam's emerging relational needs.

General principles

It has been axiomatic within psychoanalysis from the beginning that the unconscious of the patient and that of the therapist can communicate directly "without passing through consciousness" (Freud, 1915b, p. 194). (See also Freud, 1912b; Ferenczi, 1915; Bass, 2015). Bion's (1962) interpersonalization of Klein's (1946) concept of projective identification in his principle of "container/contained" introduced the idea of an unconscious intersubjective *collaboration* in the service of an infant's or patient's development—specifically the development of the capacity to process and transform raw emotional experience into thinkable, "dreamable" forms. I am broadening and individualizing Bion's vision to posit a more general unconscious collaboration through which patient and analyst work to co-create forms of understanding and relational engagement specifically and progressively fitted to each patient's total, uniquely complex, evolving therapeutic struggles, aims, and needs. These ideas also broaden Tolpin's (2002) focus on the forward edge of *the patient's* transferences and unconscious communications into an intersubjective systems construct in which not only the patient's unconscious but the "relational unconscious" (Lyons-Ruth, 1999; Gerson, 2004; Harris, 2004; Bromberg, 2011) has a forward-looking, forward-moving tendency toward progressive, more inclusive forms of fittedness (Grossmark, 2012a, b; Boston Change Process Study Group, 2013; Aron & Atlas, 2015).[3]

The analyst's unconscious subjectivity-as-analyst

Any attempted account of an intersubjective tendency toward fittedness has to begin by recognizing the central influence of our theories on our analyzing subjectivities both conscious and unconscious. Just as Lacan (1977) believed the unconscious is structured like a language, our analyzing subjectivities are structured, in part, by the "languages" of our theories, and such structuring penetrates to the unconscious level. In particular, the movement toward progressive fittedness relies on our inculcation of our theories of needed relationship—that is, how each of our theories envisions the kinds of therapeutic response or participation our patients most need, and how each analytic therapist internalizes and integrates these theories to form his unique idiom of listening, understanding, and responding. Thus, for example, my inculcation of Brandchaft's theory of pathological accommodation (Brandchaft et al., 2010) and my own theory of "the airless world" (S. Stern, 2015, In preparation) implicitly informed my processing of Celeste's life struggles. Similarly, my familiarity with Galatzer-Levy's (2009) rendering of psychoanalytic coupled oscillators and Bollas' (1987) "expressive uses of the countertransference" were some of the frames of reference that implicitly influenced my work with Sam.

In effect, each psychoanalytic theory of needed relationship is that theory's version of how to "join directionalities" with the patient in service to the patient's implicit therapeutic/developmental needs and aims. Described in slightly different terms, the inculcation of multiple theories of needed relationship helps analytic therapists develop the "receptors" necessary to sense and implement the patient's unique forward edge strivings and needs. To help illuminate how this works, consider the example of Kohut's self psychology. Really, any psychoanalytic theory could be used to illustrate the point.

For analytic therapists who became persuaded by Kohut's (1971, 1977) theory of selfobject transferences, and the importance of recognizing them as primary motivational/developmental tendencies rather than defenses against more primary drive-based conflicts, the inculcation of this theoretical position, with all of its complex ramifications for understanding the patient and the analytic process, ultimately "seeps down" into those therapists' unconscious or implicit orientation and participation. In other language, it becomes part of their operational or procedural memory-as-therapists, which, outside of conscious awareness, affects how they experience and respond to the patient and the process. This kind of internalization of theory is what Kohut (1984) had in mind when he wrote that self-psychologically oriented analysts are not inherently more empathic than analysts from other schools; rather, the self psychologist's "broadened theoretical grasp, while not altering his basic capacity for empathy, has expanded the potential range of application of this instrument of observation" (p. 84).

The same argument could be made in relation to any systematic advance in psychoanalytic theory. I believe that the more theories of psychoanalytic needed relationships an analytic clinician has internalized and synthesized, the more competent will be their unconscious or intuitive capacity to answer the question, "What does the patient need from me" with a wide range of patients, and to "move with" each patient in the full complexity of her therapeutic needs toward progressive specificity of recognition and connection. (See also Bollas, 1989, cited in Chapter 1.)

Yet, reflecting on the clinical examples of Celeste and Sam, as well as Tom (from Chapter 3), I have to conclude that there's more to the analyst's unconscious subjectivity-as-analyst than his trained unconscious recognition capacities grounded in theoretical learning. In Chapter 3 I argued that the achievement of progressive fittedness could not emerge simply from the analyst's *intention* to find increasingly fitted understandings and relational responses. Rather, it requires a paradoxical or dialectical orientation, which *both* seeks progressive fittedness *and at the same time* participates without intention; or, to state it positively, the analyst participates with an intention always to be exercising certain unique forms of analytic freedom. One such freedom derives from Bion's (1967, 1970) injunction to approach the analytic process free of memory and desire—that is, with a radical openness to that which has not yet been perceived or understood. A second is the freedom to speak or act in improvised, emergent ways in response to the unique character and exigencies of the current analytic situation (Winnicott, 1949; Symington, 1983; Bollas, 1987; Mitchell, 1988; Ehrenberg, 1992; Hoffman, 1998; S. Stern, 2009c—Chapter 6, in this volume). My emergent thought with Sam that I could sense "no author" behind his stories is an example of the first type of freedom. It emerged from the months-long tension of holding my discomfort with our coupled oscillator without knowing what to do about it, but feeling I had to do something. It did not arrive through intentional, directed thought that I was aware of, or through empathy and introspection. It came from some unconscious "place" of undirected thought—an invention born of necessity. Likewise, my instantaneous decision to share with Tom (from Chapter 3) my experience of "feeling alone in our relationship" in response to his insult, and fear of retaliation, is an example of exercising the second type of freedom—the freedom to *act* spontaneously in response to the unique contours and exigencies of the current analytic situation, often in the context of enactments.

These two kinds of analytic freedom—one having to do with apprehension and unconscious processing, the other with relational responsiveness—point to a form of unconscious participation and creativity necessary for leaps to new, more powerful and inclusive forms of fittedness that are needed but had not yet been thought or "dreamed" (Ogden, 2009). Ogden and Gabbard (2010), following and extending Bion (1962), wrote that:

> We view the analytic process as an experience in which the patient is helped to dream with the analyst the patient's previously undreamable experience (Bion, 1962; Ogden, 2004, 2005, 2009) and, in so doing, help the patient more fully dream himself into existence.
>
> (p. 541)

This is one way to think about the unconscious processes that led to my epiphany with Sam and my spontaneous emotional revelation to Tom.

These interventions seem to have emerged from a form of unconscious processing akin to dream work, where the unconscious work is prompted by some principle of analytic *necessity* (see below)—a felt tension in the current analytic situation, as experienced by the analyst, calling for the introduction of a new, needed element that addresses or meets that tension.

Winnicott offers another vertex through which to view these processes. The first statement in his brief paper on "The Aims of Psycho-Analytical Treatment" (1962) was: "In doing psycho-analysis I aim at keeping alive" (p. 166). As we know from some of his other writings (e.g., 1949, 1969), "keeping alive" had a complex meaning for Winnicott: It meant "surviving" any form of "destructiveness" or felt negation of the analyst's subjectivity, agency, or freedom to function as the patient's analyst, which arose uniquely in any given case, often associated with more primitive (pre-subjective and pre-intersubjective) modes of psychic functioning. Winnicott believed that the analyst had to do what was necessary to stay alive in the face of this kind of psychic threat in order to continue to be of use to the patient. This would be another way of understanding what developed in the intersubjective situations with both Sam and Tom. The key interventions I have described each restored forms of psychic aliveness and freedom that were being threatened.

Non-linear systemic factors

Although both Bion and Winnicott were some of the first analytic thinkers to theorize analytic dyads as relational systems—each, in different ways, finding that *unconscious cooperation* between patient and analyst was essential to a productive analytic process—they thought of the crucial analytic functions they discovered as residing primarily "in" the analyst. By contrast, Sander's theory of a dyad's movement toward progressive fittedness grows out of our contemporary intersubjective systems sensibility. Although he never directly applied this sensibility to the analytic process in a way comparable to his formulations regarding mother-infant dyads, the question I have raised about an intersubjective tendency toward fittedness invites such a systems-oriented analysis. Coburn (2014) has clarified that, from a complexity theory perspective, nothing that happens in an analytic relationship can be attributed solely to either the patient or the analyst. All happenings are understood as reflecting the self-organizing tendency of the system as a whole, and the causal "credit" for any change is thought of as "distributed" among all sub-components of the system. This systemic understanding of the change process implies the principle of *autocatalysm* as a property of non-linear systems. Coburn defines autocatalysm as the assumption that *every analytic dyad, viewed as a complex system, generates its own unique agents of change* (2014, Kindle Edition, Introduction, "Attitudes": Attitude 4). This principle or assumption is in obvious harmony with the core assumptions of this book. My concept of needed relationship, and Sander's concepts of fittedness, and specificity of recognition and connection, all suggest that the "agents of change" are always unique and specific to each analytic dyad, and emerge on an ongoing basis through the collaboration of patient and analyst in the context of their particular analytic field.

The principle of autocatalysm suggests that whatever accounts for the tendency of the system to move toward progressive fittedness must be understood as an emergent property of the system-as-a-whole rather than as a function of the analyst's capacities alone. My hypothesis of an *intersubjective* tendency toward fittedness, implies that both patient and therapist participate in this forward movement in a way that is comparable to (though far more complex than) the spontaneous choreography of Sander's father and baby daughter caught on video. In trying to imagine exactly how this hypothesized intersubjective/systemic tendency might be operating in the sequences I have described from the treatments of Tom, Celeste, and Sam, I can think of at least two levels of analysis at which to investigate it: one that concerns the system's "motivation" to *reach toward* progressive fittedness; the other concerning the processes through which progressive fittedness is *actually achieved.*

Level 1. The first level of analysis is that of *motivational interaction.* Of course, it is true at a descriptive level that both the patient and the therapist are possessed of multiple, complex, often conflicting motivations in relation to each other, themselves, and the work of therapy and that these complex motivations are constantly evolving and shifting as a function of each party's sensitivity and reactivity to current conditions, both in their own lives and within the analytic field. As analytic therapists, we consider it part of our job to be aware of as much of this interactive motivational complexity as possible. But amid all this complexity, I am positing a *central motivational tendency* expressed as a mutual *reaching* toward progressive specificity in both recognition and connection, which constitutes the analytic equivalent to the motivations we assume underlie the miraculously coordinated behavior of the father and baby in Sander's video sequence. On the patient's side it is the implicit *forward edge strivings and longings*, assumed to be present at all times, even in the midst of seemingly trailing-edge enactments and other difficulties, which motivate and constitute her unconscious collaboration. In the broadest terms, the patient's forward-edge participation is synonymous with her simply doing her job of being an engaged patient; in Bionian terms, it is the job of bringing the uncontained to the analytic process for potential containment. On the analyst's side it is *the impulse to heal psychoanalytically* (see Chapter 1) that provides the core motivation to always be reaching for progressively fitted understandings and forms of engagement.

In the case of Celeste's first session, her forward edge striving took the manifest form of narrating her struggles and anxieties as best she understood them, and, less consciously, was present in her unformulated need to have her life-long experience of aloneness recognized and empathically (really, at a deeper level, lovingly) responded to. And my impulse to heal was evident not only in my overall receptivity and processing of Celeste's story and presence but in my more specific struggle and unconscious work, trying to cope with and use my ambivalent feelings of recognition and aversion, to *understand and meet* Celeste in a way that was analytically comparable to the baby's tiny hand grasping the father's instinctively proffered finger.

There can be significant complexities at this level of analysis. Being stuck with Sam in our months-long coupled oscillator is a case in point. Sam was highly motivated to come to his sessions and engage with me in the way that he did—telling me stories, enjoying my attentive appreciation, engaging in light-hearted spontaneous joking and playing, and hugging me on the way out. It seemed to be only me who felt there was something missing, something not happening. So, how might we think about Sam's forward-edge motivation in this situation? It seemed to be half-present, but what about the other half? Something was missing—an example of what Peltz (2012) calls "the absent." Now, in retrospect, we can see that a core part of Sam's motivation wasn't exactly missing—it was present but developmentally arrested at a very early age—that of an overwhelmed, dissociated 3-year-old who has just lost his mother and has no other adult to attune to and "find" him—no one to meet or "match" his specific traumatized state, and thus no basis or intersubjective process for establishing containment or agency in relation to his overwhelming affects.

I wouldn't say that my unconscious analyzing subjectivity could perceive this as the fully formed narrative I was later able to construct. But it registered a sense of directionlessness, an unease about the absent motivation, and a sense of it being my responsibility, not Sam's, to figure out what was happening and what to do about it. *That is, I must have unconsciously intuited that there was something needed that I would have to provide.* Now, in retrospect, I can see that there was an unconscious collaboration going on in this core area of motivation: Sam was obliviously enacting his dissociated, inwardly floundering, 3-year-old self, camouflaged, as it always had been, by his hyper-competent capacitor-self wherein he had become caregiver (both father and mother) to every significant other in his relational world. It took a year of my playing with him in this dissociated world before I began to crack the code of what was happening and thereby began to match the "unthought" self-state I had sensed but not yet "known" (Bollas, 1987). That breakthrough enabled Sam, for the first time, perhaps since the age of 3, to begin to "know himself as he was known" (Sander, 2008).

Level 2: A second level of systemic analysis is required to account for how an analytic therapist and patient advance from the motivational stage of *reaching for* greater fittedness to actually *achieving* it. I propose that the movement of the system toward progressive specificity of recognition and connection is governed by a principle of *necessity*, as in the phrase: "necessity is the mother of invention."

The principle of necessity

In Sander's brief commentary on the "miraculous" coordination of the father and daughter in the video clip as they co-create the calming touch that enables the baby to fall asleep, he wrote:

> Are we looking at some principle of wholeness—that is, building on an underlying principle of specificity in time, place, and movement that joins directionalities between component systems—a joining that is necessary to construct coherent wholeness in a "system" that can be said to "live"?
>
> (2008, pp. 221–222)

I want to call attention to the word "necessary" in this passage—"a joining that is *necessary* to construct coherent wholeness in a 'system' that can be said to 'live.'" Although Sander understates the word, I think his use of it is significant and bears further consideration. He's suggesting that the joining of directionalities of dyadic partners (the achievement of fittedness) in asymmetrical, developmentally purposed, relational systems occurs out of necessity—such joining is necessary for the progressive achievement of desired developmental/therapeutic outcomes. I would add to this the reverse statement that in analytic dyads the principle of necessity, operating "through" the subjectivities (especially the implicit or unconscious subjectivities) of both parties, is what makes their joining of directionalities possible.

What is it in the patient that determines what dream will be dreamt, what traumatic experience will be remembered, what interactive detail will be seized upon for transferential and associative use, or what new insight will coalesce at a given point in time? Similarly, what is it in the analyst that envisions some potential developmental trajectory for a patient (Loewald, 1960), guides the analyst's reverie and thought processes as he sits listening, observing, and silently participating (Bion, 1962; Ogden, 1994, 1997), or senses how to word, time, and deliver an intervention in a way that is likely to resonate and transform? My sense is that these "choices" are all a function of the implicit *purposes* of the analytic dyad as a complex system—the largely unconscious developmental problem-solving aims and initiatives of the patient as these implicitly structure the analytic field, in conjunction with the (partially unconscious, intuitive) facilitation of those problem-solving efforts by the analyst. Analytic therapy is always a case of necessity being the mother of invention, where "invention" refers to the total coordination and co-creativity of the dyad in a given moment (i.e., the emergent yield of the particular momentary organization of all of the relevant sub-systems) in the service of aiding the patient in her fitful movement toward implicit, always-evolving, never-fully-namable, developmental/therapeutic aims.

Thus, my "choice" to share with Tom (in Chapter 3) my experience of feeling alone in our relationship; my "choice" to say to Celeste, as our first meeting was coming to an end, that I was aware of feeling like we weren't quite connecting, that I saw her feeling alone in all of the scenes of her life, and thought she must be doing something to cause that experience to be repeated; and my "choice" to share with Sam my unbidden thought that I could sense no author behind his stories—all were inspired, ultimately, by my implicit sense of the necessity of the moment. If I am right, the art of psychoanalysis might be understood, in part, as this evolved capacity to sense the *complexity and necessity* of the analytic moment as we intuit what to say next and how to say it.

The more precise statement would be that it is the therapist's implicit, subjective registration and interpretation of necessity, rather than the direct perception of some putative objective reality waiting to be recognized, which underwrites the process. Necessity, as I am imagining it, is a concept akin to Bion's (1970) **O**, or more precisely, is an aspect of **O**. If **O** refers to *what is*—the ultimate, never fully knowable, reality of the patient, the analytic situation, and the analytic moment—necessity refers to the reality of *what is needed* in the present moment of encounter. As with **O**, it can never be fully perceived or known; yet we try to orient to it and grasp it, using all of our faculties, including, as Bion (1967, 1970) emphasized, our free-floating intuition, albeit a highly educated and experienced intuition. Of course, since our experience of necessity is via our own subjectivities, conscious and unconscious, our interpretations of, and beliefs about, what is needed reflect our personal subjectivities in all of their complexity. They are thus subject to all manner of motivated bias related to: our creativity and wisdom; our implicitly held theories; and our own needs, states, and transferences. Our subjectivities are all we have, so we do the best we can to grasp *what is needed in service to the patient's implicit aims and strivings*, assisted by our theories that emphasize reflective awareness and therapeutic use of the complexities of our own subjectivities.

The principle of necessity accrues meaning and depth as one considers it from a number of different frames of reference. The following outline, summarizing some of these vertices, is offered to better triangulate the concept.

A. Sander's construct of "specificity of recognition," is derived from Weiss' (1970) principle of "matched specificities," and has Darwinian overtones. It is proposed as a principle of nature that accounts for the mysterious process through which individuals develop into coherently organized, optimally functioning complex systems within their surrounding social eco-systems. Understood within this biological/evolutionary frame, the principle of matched specificities is being proposed as the organizing form through which the more fundamental principle of necessity is actualized as developmental process. In plain language, Sander (following Weiss) is arguing that specificity of recognition and connection are *necessary* for optimal human development or, in an adult treatment context, for certain aspects of development that have been compromised in developmentally traumatized patients.

B. In the therapeutic context, the principle of necessity connects with the idea of needed relationship but by way of a complex path. The shift to a holistic model means abandoning the particular guiding assumptions embodied in any one (or even any several) of our theories—assumptions that structure our thinking and perceptions regarding the nature of what our patients struggle with, especially unconsciously, and what kinds of intervention they need from us to help them transform those struggles. It seems to me that what we are left with as we let go of particular guiding theories is the principle of necessity. By necessity, here, I mean our subjective sense of what to do next based on our current grasp of all of the interacting forces and tensions: within the patient; within ourselves in relation to the patient; between the patient and ourselves; and between the patient and his total relational world. Of course, our sense of these interacting forces and tensions is informed by all of the theories we have internalized and the complex, fluid interactions among them within our conscious and unconscious subjectivities as we engage as participant-observers. But by letting go of our theories, even as we use them, we are freer to allow more of the total system or field, in all of its dense, fluid complexity, to inform and shape our evolving sense of the complex *constellations of necessity* operating from moment to moment and session to session, which in turn better enables us to *contour* our total response to that ever-morphing system of constellations.

Thus with Celeste, as our first session evolved, necessity took the form of my determined preoccupation with my aversive countertransference as a felt interference with, but also clue to, the needed relationship we were reaching toward.

I agreed to hug Sam based on the "feel" of his request and its impact on me. My sense was to go with it. Only years later can I now speculate that Sam's developmental trauma—the loss of his mother, and any semblance of a maternal holding environment, at age 2 or 3—left him with powerful longings for physical touch, tenderness. and holding. Similarly, the nature and repetitive quality of our daily interactions—our coupled oscillator—which I also at first fell in with at the implicit level, now seems clearly to signify Sam's need for a reliably asymmetrical, unconditionally welcoming and admiring relational context, which he also, presumably, lost at a very young age.

Things became more complicated with the gradual onset of my feelings of directionlessness and therapeutic stasis: complicated in the sense that this experience of "chafing" (D.B. Stern, 2010) came not only from my experience of Sam but from my understanding of "the feel" of a productive analytic process, based on my immersion in psychoanalytic theories and decades of clinical experience. Some essential element of a productive analytic process was (or felt to me to be) absent, and was thus *in need* of attention and some kind of problem analysis. At that juncture, the constellations of necessity expanded to include not only Sam's implicitly *felt needs*, empathically sensed by me, but a more objective perception of something both Sam and our process "needed" that lay outside the realm of Sam's (even unconscious) subjectivity (Gedo, 1979).

C. The principle of necessity operates at the level of the implicit, but it is the implicit at its most complex. The implicit sensing of analytic necessity is not exactly in the same register as "implicit relational knowing" (D.N. Stern, et al., 1998; Lyons-Ruth et al., 1998), although it includes the analyst's total implicit relational knowing in the present moment of analytic interaction and choice. It is closer to the register that contemporary Bionian authors call the analytic field (Peltz, 2012; Peltz & Goldberg, 2013; Ferro & Civitarese, 2013), although they have no explicit construct of necessity. We might say that the sensing of necessity occurs within the analyst's relationship not only to the patient (intersubjective register) but to the analytic field as a kind of third (containing) presence. The analyst infers or grasps necessity from all that is going on in the analytic field, taking the measure of the current confluence of many elements and integrating them into an expressive whole, which, if recurrently successful over the course of treatment, renders the patient more whole.

D. The principle of necessity, as I intend it, addresses the conceptual gap in non-linear dynamic systems theory identified in Chapter 2 regarding the relationship between the complex system of the analytic dyad and the complex system "going on" within the analyst's analyzing subjectivity. We now understand that the analytic therapist—everything he experiences, thinks, says, and does—is fully contextualized by his embeddedness in the intersubjective system of the dyad: Everything is emergent from the ongoing life of the system as a whole. At the same time, he occupies a position of navigational and transformational responsibility for the patient and the process: in other words, responsibility for the movement of the system in analytically productive directions, or toward what Sander (2008) describes as "coherent wholeness." This paradox or conundrum seems unique to therapeutic systems wherein, unlike parent-child systems, the contemporary analyst requires expertise in, and seeks reflective awareness of, the workings of the system as a whole so as to be able to shepherd the system and its process analytically. In a systems theory frame, *the analyst is in the paradoxical position of functioning as the container (Bion, 1962) for the system that contains him.* Viewed in this way, the history of psychoanalytic theories and ideas could be understood as an evolving set of guidelines for the complex task of occupying this paradoxical position.

Necessity is the principle, or at least one important principle, that takes account of and, in a sense, exploits this paradoxical position. As an integral, fully embedded "component" of the system, the analyst has intimate, first-hand experience of the complex *constellations of necessity* "bearing down" on (and expressed through) the patient-analyst system moment-to-moment in the form of felt (sensed) tensions. At the same time, through his conscious and unconscious processing of these tensions, he is in a position to transform them into needed forms of understanding and engagement—that is, to address the patient's complex aims and needs (experience of necessity) that originally brought her to treatment and remain throughout the primary driver of her participation, and thus of the analytic system and field.

E. Although necessity is always gauged and acted upon in the present analytic moment, part of what is being taken into account in that moment is the temporal dimension of the process as channeled through the analyst's understanding and participation. I wrote about this in connection with my 9-year treatment of Linda described in Chapter 1. In that case, necessity was operating on both sides of my paradoxical stance. My active efforts to influence Linda's commitment to coming more regularly over a sufficient length of time grew out of a complex sense I developed of what she (Linda in particular) would *need* to do (in the future) in order to realize her core therapeutic aims. At the same time, it was equally *necessary* for me to recognize and respect her anxieties about such a commitment, and thus to engage with her (in the present moment) in a fundamentally accepting, empathic, emancipatory (non-controlling) fashion—that is, conveying that I did not need her to be different from the way she already was and needed to be. As we deconstruct this complex stance, we can see necessity operating in my efforts to get Linda to change, in my acceptance of her exactly as she was, and in the unique qualities of language and voice we co-created over time to express and contain the paradox—the "push and pull" of necessity—and render both sides actionable. We might say that necessity took into account what was needed, what was possible, and the potential trajectory over time through which what was possible needed to evolve in order to make what was needed possible. And these "bits of necessity" were only a small (though prominent) part of the infinitely complex "system of necessity" operating moment-to-moment, affecting my clinical choices at both conscious and implicit levels.

F. The principle of necessity generates tensions that help keep the analyst oriented toward that which is not yet known or understood. Such tensions were clearly operating in my work with Sam, for example, during the long period of my unease, confusion, and uncertainty stemming from the sense of directionlessness. The unbidden thought that cracked open our circular coupled oscillator and set in motion a cascade of transformative dialogue felt relieving, exciting and productive because it had "cracked the code" of the enigma generated by the particular form necessity had taken during the period of uncertainty, thereby rapidly reducing (though not completely eliminating) the felt tension of necessity.

G. The imprint of necessity can be seen (and felt) in the later stages of good-enough treatments when the analytic couple has achieved highly evolved, complex forms of fittedness, which are known to have both produced and emerged from the many transformations responsible for the system's and the patient's greater competence, or to use Sander's word, greater "wholeness." In the later stages of treatment the sense of "knowing oneself as one is known" is deeply felt by both parties, to the point where needed understandings and relational gestures occur with greater speed and ease than at earlier stages. This doesn't mean that all is settled that needs to be settled, or that there still aren't blind spots, either old or new, that *need* to be recognized and addressed in order for further transformation-toward-termination to occur. One can assume that necessity is still present until the patient has terminated, hopefully in whatever way she or he *needed* to. I am reminded here of a patient who, after all of the struggles that had brought him to therapy and organized our years-long work together seemed to be well understood and worked through, continued coming to sessions for five or six more months, sitting in almost complete silence. The feeling in the room during this period was one of ease and peace. The need for this additional time was never completely understood, but, as best the patient could express it, involved a process of inner integration which apparently still required my presence.

H. As will be explored more fully in the closing chapter of this book, the waning of necessity is often marked by the gradual arrival and deepening of a sense of *peace* relative to the struggles for which the patient sought analytic treatment. Necessity in an analytic context involves tensions of one sort or another—tensions set in motion by the patient's struggles and aims and the analyst's struggles in relation to the patient—as these come to organize the analytic field as a complex system. These tensions prompt our efforts (conscious and unconscious) to recognize, meet, and transform the patient's struggles, which, if successful, occasion the arrival of a sense of peace relative to those struggles. This sense of peace is initially established and expanded *intersubjectively*. But in the end we hope that it can be carried by the patient when no longer in the physical presence of the analyst. I view the arrival and consolidation of the sense of relative peace as the analytic equivalent of the baby in Sander's video falling asleep, having gotten the assistance she needed from the father's magic touch and the mysterious principle of necessity operating through both of them as they reached for each other in tandem.

Notes

1 One of the purposes of Sullivan's "detailed inquiry" was to detect incongruities in the patient's narrative: points where, because of the patient's selective inattention and parataxic distortions, the story wasn't fitting together. Sullivan would tactfully but pointedly challenge these "convenient fictions" so as to get an "adequate account" and, in the process, begin to invite and support the truer (but dissociated) cause-and-effect interpersonal history and its associated affects. Like Winnicott, Sullivan's instinctive capacity to discern these points of ill-fittedness required that he "have in his bones a theory of emotional development of the child and of the relationship of the child to the environmental factors."

2 According to Galatzer-Levy, the original and prototypic example of a coupled oscillator was the spontaneous synchronization of the pendulum motions of two wall clocks, first observed in the seventeenth century. "Oscillators are said to be coupled if they are connected in some way . . . The resonant vibrations of piano strings, the coupling of two weighted springs by a rubber band, the coupling of two neurons through connections in a neural network, and the back and forth movement of dancers, all are usefully conceptualized as coupled oscillators" (2009, p. 988). One of the points of Galatzer-Levy's paper is that an analyst and patient, functioning as a non-linear dynamic system, can evolve powerfully therapeutic forms and patterns of connection through processes that take place outside the area of linear, cognitively grounded, cause-and-effect relationships posited in psychoanalytic theories of therapeutic action.

3 See the Appendix for a comparison between the BCPSG (2013), Grossmark (2012a, b), Aron and Atlas (2015), and the model presented in this chapter.

Chapter 5

Understanding and engagement in the analytic process

> We contend that all show involves tell, and all tell involves show. Words and actions, remembering and repeating, association and enactment, interpretation and non-interpretive interventions are all transformations of each other. They all contain and rely upon one another, and should be thought of dialectically rather than dichotomously.
>
> (Lewis Aron, 2012)[1]

The relational model, in the broad, historical sense that Greenberg and Mitchell (1983) had in mind when they first introduced the term, has brought with it an increasing appreciation, and theoretical embrace, of the relational factors involved in the psychoanalytic process. Every major "relational model" theorist has introduced new ways of thinking about these relational factors, which grow out of the theorist's total paradigm that includes the nature of mind, development, psychopathology, the analytic process, and therapeutic action. Most of these theorists have been careful not to say or imply that *relational engagement* means abandoning the emphasis Freud placed on *understanding* as a central objective and curative mechanism of psychoanalytic treatment. Winnicott (1969), for example, in the introduction to his paper on "The Use of an Object," famously wrote:

> . . . it is only in recent years that I have become able to wait and wait for the natural evolution of the transference arising out of the patient's growing trust in the psychoanalytic technique and setting, and to avoid breaking up this natural process by making interpretations. It will be noticed that I am talking about the making of interpretations and not

> about interpretations as such. It appals me to think how much deep change I have prevented or delayed in patients *in a certain classification category* by my personal need to interpret. If only we can wait, the patient arrives at understanding creatively and with immense joy, and I now enjoy this joy more that I used to enjoy the sense of having been clever.
>
> (p. 86; emphasis in the original)

In other words, the central importance of understanding and interpretation is not being eschewed; it is being re-situated within a larger relational context defined, in Winnicott's case, by such factors as the creation of a holding environment, non-impingement, the winning of trust, an implicit expectation regarding the patient's self-analytic motivations and capacities, the analyst's own sense of joy and aliveness in the process, and, in general, the establishment of relational conditions conducive to the emergence of understanding and self-understanding as an aspect of analytic growth.

As in so many areas of analytic discourse, Winnicott's thinking here opened a potential space in both clinical theory and analytic practice—a potential space that made possible the (r)evolution that became relational psychoanalysis. In his deceptively personal, homespun prose, Winnicott introduced an expansion of the nature and role of psychoanalytic understanding to include *understanding of the relational conditions—i.e., the kinds of relational engagement, environment, and atmosphere—thought necessary for the emergence of understanding, and ultimately, for the patient's psychological growth.* This shift frees the analyst's efforts to understand from the classical straightjacket within which verbal interpretation was the sole, or at least privileged, vehicle for expressing that understanding. Rather, a new space has opened up wherein the analyst's understanding may tell her that what could be most helpful for a given patient at a given point in treatment is some non-verbal relational response that better meets the patient's need of the moment, or better serves the creation of an analytic process that is optimally facilitative of the patient's overall growth process. In short, in this new analytic potential space, theoretically informed relational engagement is thought to *reflect*, not forsake, understanding (both general and case-specific) and is thought to be an essential factor contributing to a patient's experience of feeling understood.

Yet, with the progression of relational theory from its mid-century pioneers (Balint, Fairbairn, Winnicott, Sullivan, Bion, Kohut, Loewald, Racker, Searles) to the profusion of relational, intersubjective, constructivist, and hermeneutic perspectives that have emerged during the past three decades, the theorized relationship between understanding and relational engagement has become increasingly complex and murky. In the present chapter I sort through some of this complexity as background for articulating my own current integration of these two co-occurring, interpenetrating dimensions of analytic interaction. The essence of my position is stated in Principle #3 of the meta-theory of needed relationships (see Introduction):

> Progressive fittedness involves progressive *understanding*; progressive shaping of the ways we learn to *listen, process, and speak* with each patient; and progressive fittedness in the *forms and qualities of relational engagement* that emerge in each treatment. Understanding ("truth") and relational engagement are viewed as inseparable and as operating synergistically. In Sander's (2008) language, achieving progressive fittedness in the service of either a child's or patient's psychological growth requires both *specificity of recognition* and *specificity of connection.*

As the opening quote from Aron (2012) indicates, I am not alone in thinking about the analytic process in this way. Undoubtedly, many relational analysts and therapists now adopt some version of this holistic view of analytic engagement. But it is far from universally accepted. Different theorists, and schools of analytic thought, still privilege one side of the dialectic over the other. Thus, it is useful to look at the evolution of relational thinking about these issues in order to better understand the diversity and murkiness that still prevails.

Because of the length of this chapter, necessitated by the scope of the topic and its centrality as an issue in much contemporary relational analytic theorizing, I will briefly outline the sequence of sub-topics (sections) here and summarize the major points of the chapter in its concluding section.

1 I begin by examining some of the influential relational formulations regarding the relationship between *understanding* and *relational engagement* in therapeutic action and transformation. Theorists covered include Kohut, Mitchell, Weiss and Sampson, Stolorow, contemporary Bionian authors, Ehrenberg, Hoffman, Aron, Harris, and Bacal.
2 I examine in depth the recent trend in analytic theory, influenced by mother-infant research, neuroscience, and cognitive psychology, privileging the role of "implicit" (un-symbolized, non-verbal) relational processes *over* "explicit," interpretive communications in therapeutic action. Using a clinical vignette, I argue that the issues here are more complex than this literature has recognized, and that a more holistic view is called for. Among authors extrapolating from mother-infant research to adult treatment, I find Sander's thinking to be the most holistic.
3 I present my own synthesis, illustrated by an "ordinary" clinical example.

A selective historical review and analysis

Kohut

Taking Kohut as a somewhat arbitrary starting point, his struggle with this tension seems emblematic of the murkiness that the late-mid-century relational models introduced. Initially, Kohut (1959) viewed his formulation of the empathic-introspective listening stance as an advance in the data-gathering, observational capacities of the analyst. In a revolutionary, paradigm changing move, he recognized that a consistent focus on seeking to understand the patient's subjective experience from the patient's perspective (as opposed to seeking to discern more "experience distant" dynamics described in psychoanalytic theories and meta-theories) was both a better route to the kind of understanding that was most relevant to psychoanalysts, and, because of the positive effects on the patient of feeling understood in this way, a method more likely to prompt the patient to reveal the most emotionally significant, analytically relevant "data." This aspect of Kohut's new formulations could be seen as mainly an advance in the analyst's capacities to understand. Indeed, wanting to be seen as still doing psychoanalysis, Kohut (1971, 1977, 1984) repeatedly insisted that the self-psychological analyst's job was not to gratify or meet patients' selfobject needs but to empathically understand and validate them. However, in his last formulations of the issue (Kohut, 1982, 1984), dramatized famously in his (1982) clinical vignette in which he allowed a regressed patient on the couch to hold two of his fingers, he acknowledged that the analyst's empathic responsiveness was also a form of relational engagement with the properties of a corrective emotional experience. In some of his final words on the topic, Kohut (1984) wrote that one of the cumulative yields of a successful self-psychological analysis was the patient's "increasing realization that, contrary to his experiences in childhood, the sustaining echo of empathic resonance is indeed available in this world" (p. 78). One can sense Kohut struggling with the conundrum of understanding and engagement, never quite reaching a clear conclusion about it.

It should be said, however, that although Kohut struggled with the question of what *the analyst did and should do* to promote the "restoration of the self" (Kohut, 1977), he recognized that on the patient's side of things, far more was going on relationally than simply the experience of the analyst's empathic understanding. In the other truly revolutionary part of his thinking, Kohut recognized that certain patients required new relational experiences with the analyst via the selfobject transferences: mirroring, idealizing, and twinship. He believed that with an analyst functioning in an empathic/interpretive (i.e., fairly traditional) mode, but armed with an in-depth understanding of the psychology of the self that would enable the analyst to *accept* the selfobject transferences as expressing legitimate needs, such patients would experience the analyst as serving needed relational/developmental functions comparable (though not identical) to those served by the healthy-enough parents of young children. Significantly, Kohut believed that, in order for analysts to perform these functions, they had to be prepared to engage in one particular form of relational behavior that departed from the traditional psychoanalytic stance: They needed to acknowledge, and when appropriate, take responsibility and apologize for, the effects of their own unintentional empathic errors and/or treatment of the patient that had been experienced as retraumatizing. This occasional ownership of responsibility, in conjunction with the analyst's accepting attitude and accurate-enough interpretations of the impact of the analyst's behavior on the patient's self-states, were the main relational activities the analyst needed to engage in in order to support the patient's new relational experience of the analyst-as-selfobject. Yet, this one move toward explicit relationality was historically significant in that it brought the analyst in as a human being who, with the best of intentions, could make mistakes that had real consequences; but who also, hopefully, had the maturity, sensitivity, and ethical motivation to acknowledge them and repair the damage.

"Developmental arrest" theories

Both Winnicott and Kohut were contributors to a paradigm shift in late-mid-twentieth century analytic thought that moved psychoanalysis in the direction of viewing the analyst as a kind of *reparenting figure* or *new object* (Fairbairn, 1958) who, in diverse ways, exerted a positive developmental influence, not only as a transference creation of the patient but as a co-creation of the patient and analyst that included the analyst's *intention* to function in this development-facilitating way (Fairbairn, 1952, 1958; Bion, 1962; Balint, 1968; Winnicott, 1965, 1971a; Bowlby, 1975; Loewald, 1960; Kohut, 1971, 1977, 1984). Within the unique intersubjective potential space of analysis, these empathic, mirroring, idealizing, holding, containing, protective, confronting, educative, supportive, playful, loving, freeing, and other developmental functions tend to be expressed in more subtle, paradoxical, symbolically mediated forms than they are in the actual parenting of young children. But the point is that, in all of these developmental models, relational/emotional engagement was emerging as a new defining current of an optimal analytic attitude and approach—one that stood in a not-fully-formulated relationship to the traditional current emphasizing progressive understanding and dispassionate communication of the patient's truth as revealed through the analytic dialogue.

Relational theories of the 1980s

Then, beginning in the 1980s, Bollas, Mitchell, Ehrenberg, Hoffman, Aron, Benjamin, Bromberg, Davies, Pizer, and other early relationalists built on these relational trends in developmental-arrest thinking (Mitchell, 1988), and, influenced by other theoretical streams—notably the Kleinian/Bionian, existential, and Sullivanian interpersonal traditions—expanded the *kinds* of relational engagement being advocated to include more adult-to-adult forms that were not framed as analytic equivalents of parental functions. Authenticity, spontaneity, mutuality, and selective, intentional disclosure of countertransference and other personal feelings and information emerged as new relational possibilities that were shown to carry great therapeutic power in a wide range of clinical situations. These developments reflected a fully "two-person" re-envisioning of the analytic encounter in which the analyst's more personal engagement was seen to deepen the connection in ways that both expanded the content of what could be talked about and exerted a freeing and transforming influence on the patient's capacities for self-delineation and relational/emotional connection. One might say that, in the Relational model of the 1980s and 90s, the selective revelation of *the analyst's subjectivity in relation to the patient* was found not only to elicit and illuminate but also to transform the patient's psychic reality (truth) in ways that had not been possible within earlier psychoanalytic models.

The result of this theoretical (r)evolution—one that had been gaining momentum since mid-century in the developmental-arrest models—was a continuing, accelerating shift away from interpretation-leading-to-insight as the exclusive mechanism of therapeutic action and *telos* of analytic therapy (Mitchell, 1997, chapter 5). Given that the real goals of analysis were (and had always been) transformations in the patient's experience of self-in-relation-to-others, and expanded and enriched capacities for navigating both the internal-object and external-relational worlds, if new, non-interpretive forms of relational engagement led directly to such transformations, the central importance of interpretation leading to insight was called into question. Again, none of these theorists denied the importance of understanding, and many continued to view interpretation as a primary vehicle of analytic transformation (Bollas, 1987; Mitchell, 1988; Davies & Frawley, 1994). But, to say the least, the relationship between relational engagement and understanding was becoming more complex.

Since the early 1980s many theoretical variations have emerged in which these two fundamental currents in our thinking about therapeutic action have begun to be integrated in more complex and sophisticated ways.

Mitchell

Mitchell (1988, 1997) recognized that mutative interpretations were always *both* an imparting of understanding and a new relational experience, and that unless an interpretation was also *felt* as a new experience, the content of the interpretation could too easily be conscripted into the patient's *old* patterns of relating and meaning-making. But Mitchell also went "beyond interpretation" in the traditional sense by introducing a new form of verbal intervention: the analyst's struggle to "find an authentic voice" with which to speak to the analysand from within the turbulence of co-created enactments—a voice that was simultaneously a new form of relational engagement *and* a kind of interpretation of the transference-countertransference impasse.

Weiss and Sampson

Coming out of the ego-psychological tradition, Weiss and Sampson (1986) were among the first to recognize that a patient's experience of the analyst as *responding differently* than the patient's old objects in crucial ways at critical moments (thereby disconfirming the patient's "pathogenic beliefs" based on past traumas) often leads spontaneously to insight (really, an unconscious opening to formerly warded off affective experience and memory) without the analyst always having to make explicit interpretations. Their "control-mastery" theory was grounded in Freud's (1926, 1940) later thinking regarding the ego's unconscious regulation of repressions and the unconscious impulse and movement toward mastery, based on the implicit criterion of subjectively sensed safety vs. danger. Since the 1980s, Weiss and Sampson's insight has expanded to a general recognition that the felt relational context of each analytic relationship, especially the degree to which the therapist is experienced as a safe new object in the transference, exerts an enormous shaping influence on the content and quality of what emerges in the patient's verbal and implicit communications, and thus on the quality of insight and understanding that become possible.

Stolorow and collaborators

Stolorow (2006), who, along with his co-authors (Stolorow, Brandchaft, & Atwood, 1987; Stolorow & Atwood, 1992; Stolorow, Atwood, & Brandchaft, 1994; Stolorow, Atwood, & Orange, 2002), recontextualized many of Kohut's ideas within a contemporary intersubjective, hermeneutic frame, has stressed that the chief function of psychoanalysis is to provide a "relational home" for the patient's formerly unrecognized, unvalidated, and unintegrated, "prereflective" affective experience. The implication is that only insofar as the patient experiences the therapist's attitude as truly *welcoming* can an optimal context be established for the illumination, symbolization (putting into words), and integration of the patient's "experiential world." One can sense, however, that Stolorow and his associates continued to straddle the same fence that Kohut did in this regard. They regarded an authentically welcoming attitude, sustained empathic-introspective inquiry, and the analytic function of putting words to emotional experience, as the primary forms of relational engagement our patients need; or at least they were the main forms they wrote about. Stolorow (1994) acknowledged a role for "affective responsiveness" as a separate curative factor, and, like Kohut, recognized that the experience of being understood can in itself constitute a new corrective relational experience. He also believed, following Kohut, that when patients were experiencing the "developmental (selfobject) dimension of the transference," the analyst needed to do little beyond empathic listening, inquiry, and welcoming for the patient to experience the analytic engagement as a new relational experience (Stolorow, Brandchaft, & Atwood, 1987). But the vast majority of his and his associates' theorizing pertained to the empathic apprehension, understanding, and articulation of the patient's experiential world. As they characterized it:

> Psychoanalysis . . . is a dialogic exploration of a patient's experiential world, conducted with awareness of the unavertable contribution of the analyst's experiential world to the ongoing exploration. Such empathic-introspective inquiry *seeks understanding* of what the patient's world feels like, of what emotional and relational experiences it includes, often relentlessly, and what it assiduously excludes and precludes. It *seeks comprehension* of the network of convictions, the rules or principles that prereflectively organize the patient's world and keep the patient's experiencing confined to its frozen horizons and limiting perspectives. By *illuminating* such principles in a dialogic process and by grasping their life-historical origins, psychoanalysis aims to expand the patient's experiential horizons, thereby opening up the possibility of an enriched, more complex, and more flexible emotional life.
>
> (Stolorow, et al., 2002, p. 46; emphasis added)

And in a more recent distillation, Stolorow (2006) wrote:

> I have become convinced that it is in the process of somatic-symbolic integration, the process through which emotional experience comes into language, that the sense of being is born.
>
> (p. 240)

While these quotes constitute an eloquent and comprehensive account of the pursuit of psychoanalytic understanding, and a major advance on the classical model of objectively rendered interpretation leading to insight, the analytic tools Stolorow and his coauthors employed represented an epistemologically more contemporary, intersubjective embodiment of the principle of *understanding* as the chief engine of analytic transformation, and thus remained only half the story.[2]

In his most recent writings, Stolorow has expanded his thinking on these issues, moving closer to a recognition of the importance of relational engagement, especially in the analytic treatment of trauma (Stolorow, 2014). He has come to the understanding that traumatized patients require a form of analyst participation he calls "emotional dwelling." In emotional dwelling the analyst not only welcomes the patient's dissociated and repressed affects, he accompanies the patient in an undiluted encounter with (a not-turning-away-from) the overwhelmingly painful affects and the associated experience of self-in-relational-to-world that are the legacy of trauma. Stolorow clearly intends emotional dwelling as a form of relational engagement. However, it is only one particular form that grows out of his theory of trauma. Thus, he still seems to stop short (at least in his theoretical writing) of recognizing that relational engagement can take many forms depending on the unique process and needs that are emergent within each analytic relationship as it evolves over time.

Contemporary Bionian theorists

Coming from a very different theoretical tradition than Kohut and Stolorow, contemporary followers of Bion end up in a surprisingly similar position with regard to the prioritization of the analyst's understanding functions, broadly defined. While there is no way to do justice to this complex and evolving theory (with many contemporary variations) in a terse summary, I think it is fair to say that this large and rapidly growing international community of analysts and theorists follow Bion (1962) in their assumption that serious forms of psychopathology are mainly disorders of "thinking"—specifically, breakdowns in the essential capacity for unconscious processing (thinking, dreaming, reverie, "alpha function") through which raw emotional experience becomes transformed into "thinkable" experience now useable for growth purposes (Ogden, 1994, 1997, 2009; Ogden & Gabbard, 2010; Ferro, 2005; Ferro & Civitarese, 2013; Peltz, 2012; Peltz & Goldberg, 2013; Neri, 2009; Symington, 2012).

Ogden and Gabbard (2010) describe the *telos* of this model as follows: "The aim of psychoanalysis . . . is truth-focused (focused on helping the patient learn from and become the truth of his emotional experience) . . . " (p. 534). While this current of thought derives historically from Freud's and Klein's one-person focus on "objective" analytic understanding leading to interpretation and insight, these contemporary, post-Bionian iterations embed the analyst in a two-person, intersubjective matrix and offer therapeutic narratives in which understanding emerges, not from detached, objective observation, but from the subjective experience of participation in the vicissitudes of the transference-countertransference dynamic, and the intersubjective field more generally (Ogden, 1994, 1997; Peltz, 2012; Peltz & Goldberg, 2013; Ferro & Civitarese, 2013). Specifically, understanding emerges from the analyst's capacity to observe, process (through reverie), and reflect on her subjective experience within "the intersubjective analytic third" or "analytic field."

While the contemporary Bionian version of intersubjectivity is very different from Stolorow's intersubjective systems model, the analyst's containing functions in the Bionian model and Stolorow et al.'s sustained empathic inquiry leading to illumination of the patient's experiential world, both pretty much confine the analyst's relational engagement to functions having to do with understanding, thinking, the processing of the patient's unbearable feelings, and the illumination of the patient's psychic reality. Also, while both of these models recognize the analyst's inevitable susceptibility to becoming caught up in problematic relational scenarios (in the transference-countertransference dynamic), potentially leading to impasse, both models have more faith in the analyst's ability to catch, process, "decenter" from, and transform such enactments through intentional self-observation and reflective work (Bion's "second look") than does the American Relational school. Analysts in the latter tradition argue that because enactments, by their nature, involve the analyst's unconscious participation (relational engagement), the analyst can never be fully confident in her ability to "see" and transcend them (Hoffman, 1983, 1998; D.B. Stern, 2010, 2013a, b). Accordingly, given the analyst's irreducibly subjective participation in all aspects of the process, especially enactments, Relationalists have theorized that the best "way out" of many enactments is often "through" the analyst's "finding a voice" with which to authentically express her subjective experience of what is happening (her current "self state") in a direct, but non-critical, non-blaming way—a voice that simultaneously *expresses and holds* her emotional experience and participation as an "analytic object" (Green, 1975) to be reflected on and used in the service of deepening understanding and connection (Bollas, 1987; Mitchell, 1988, 1997; Ehrenberg, 1992; Hoffman, 1998; Bromberg, 2011).

A blind spot in Bionian field theory

Some contemporary "Bionian field theorists," comparing their approach with contemporary Relational theory, privilege the analytic field over the real analytic relationship itself as the primary system of interest, and source of analytic data (Ferro & Civitarese, 2013; Peltz & Goldberg, 2013). While the intersubjective relationship is viewed as an important vertex (frame of reference; point of entry) to which the analyst's attention may be drawn, and through which analytic data is processed, these authors emphasize the total psycho-sensory apprehension of all that is happening, with maximum openness to whatever emerges or impinges on awareness (especially the edges of awareness). Thus reverie, sensory-somatic states, fantasy, memory, affects, impulses, images, inklings of both difficulty and promise, the emergence of "selected facts," pulls on the analyst's attention, aversions, and senses of something missing, are what the analyst is trying (in as relaxed and alert a state as possible) to register and process (e.g., Ogden, 1994, 1997; Peltz, 2012; Peltz & Goldberg, 2013). This orientation aligns with the Bionian assumption that many (perhaps all) psychoanalytic patients' suffer primarily from difficulties in "thinking" and "dreaming" their emotional experience (Ogden & Gabbard, 2010); thus the analyst's primary job is to be able register, think, "dream," and ultimately communicate in useable form the (mostly out-of-awareness) emotional reality of what is occurring within the analytic field. They seem to view this processing function as outside of, or superordinate to, "real" happenings in the intersubjective analytic relationship, and "external reality" more generally (Ferro & Civitarese, 2013).

This model of the analyst's participation and function derives from Bion's (1962) theory of *container/contained* and the analyst's capacity for *reverie* and *alpha function*. Contemporary Bionian theorists thus argue that the analyst's capacities for unconscious apprehension and unconscious processing of emotional reality, and the interpretations or "narrations" that emerge from this processing, *as opposed to relational engagement*, are the primary engine of therapeutic action. The blind spot here is that container/contained *is* a form of relational engagement—one that falls in the same general category as the various analytic functions identified in the other developmental theories of the late-mid-twentieth century, such as Winnicott's holding and Kohut's selfobject functions. Like these other relational functions, container/contained is understood to be needed because of the mother's failure to have adequately performed this function for the patient as an infant and young child. Once it is recognized that *containment* is a form of real relationship, it becomes clear that *it is a real relationship that carries the therapeutic action*, and the question immediately arises: Why would one assume that containment is *the only* form of real relationship that is occurring or the only form that carries therapeutic action? Rather, it seems evident that there is always a real relationship going on, that that real relationship is in a constant state of flux (just as the analytic field is), that many other relational possibilities and engagements (some conscious and intentional, some not) are occurring as part of this relational flux, and that at least some of these carry therapeutic action.

Ehrenberg

Among the early Relational theorists, the author who, in my view, articulated the most fully realized integration of these two currents in contemporary analytic thought was Ehrenberg (1992). However, her ideas about this have not been sufficiently appreciated or incorporated into the Relational theoretical mainstream. Here is Ehrenberg's most succinct statement of her position on this topic:

> My view is that the combination of a rigorous analytic process and a vital, personal, affective engagement is crucial and that either without the other is insufficient. I believe it is the *integration* of both, and their operating not in alternation but in actual combination, as each becomes the condition for the other, that is essential and definitive. The integration of the affective and the analytic gives each more scope. Either alone could not be carried as far analytically as each can be when it is combined with the other.
>
> (pp. 66–67)

This deceptively straightforward formulation, and Ehrenberg's 1992 book illustrating it with many diverse clinical examples, capture much of what I think of as a holistic approach to the relationship between understanding and engagement in the analytic process. Mitchell, in his 1997 review and appreciation of the American interpersonal tradition, recognized Ehrenberg as an important contributor to that tradition, but characterized her contribution as primarily in the area of countertransference disclosure (pp. 91–92). I would argue that, as the above quote testifies, her clinical and theoretical vision was much broader and subtler than this. But because of the way her work was reductively characterized, these broader implications have not been fully absorbed into the Relational theoretical canon. Ehrenberg applies her conceptual synthesis in her particular way. Engagement for her means a very active, direct, personal expressiveness, and a preference for verbally naming, and opening up for exploration, any nascent enactment as soon as she becomes aware of it. That is her authentic idiom (Bollas, 1987) of participation, and it seems to have worked extremely well for her and her patients. But the general principles she articulated regarding the integration of "analytic rigor" (in the service of progressive understanding), and personal affective engagement, can potentially be adapted by any analytic therapist within her own idiom of participation.

Hoffman

The other early Relational theorist whose thinking "created a space" for the technical integration of disciplined analytic exploration (leading to understanding) and more relationally engaged personal expressiveness was Hoffman (1998). He approached such issues *dialectically*—that is, with a sensibility in which two seemingly opposing principles are seen as having a complex relationship to each other, and thus held in mind not as an "either/or" binary but as a "both/and" dialectical tension. Hoffman described a number of such dialectics, but the best known (which provided the title of his 1998 book) was the dialectic of ritualized, disciplined (i.e., more traditional) analytic inquiry vs. spontaneous, personal expressiveness leading to a sense of shared humanity and more intimate, personal connection. In the 1994 paper in which Hoffman first presented his dialectical approach, the case example he chose—one of his analytic control cases—was a patient who, for understandable personal historical reasons, stubbornly resisted traditional analytic dialogue in which the analyst waits and listens, the patient initiates self-reflective associations, and the analyst interprets. Instead, she seemed to need Hoffman to deviate from the traditional role and engage with her in more practical problem-solving and, at times, more personally real emotional exchange. What Hoffman came to realize was that, if he stubbornly tried to hold out for reflective dialogue, little happened; whereas if he, at times, yielded to the patient's demand for his more personal, down-to-earth responsiveness, she *then became interested* in looking more reflectively at her own process. I can't do justice here to Hoffman's complex analysis of the relational cross-currents he saw operating in his negotiations with this patient. But the case and his handling of it, like many of Ehrenberg's (1992) case examples, vividly demonstrated the complex, case-specific inter-relationship between understanding and emotional engagement, and how a patient's interest in self-understanding often *follows from* the enactive co-creation of needed relational conditions.[3]

Aron and Harris

The post-millennial writings of a number of Relational authors, especially Aron (2012; Aron & Starr, 2013) and Harris (2009), have carried forward and expanded Hoffman's dialectical sensibility, taking aim at binary oppositions of all kinds, including the binary of analytic understanding vs. relational engagement. The quote from Aron (2012) that begins this chapter succinctly and eloquently expresses this sensibility, as does the following passage from Harris (2009) in which, referencing earlier work by Aron and herself (1997), she elaborates her own characterization of recent trends in Relational thinking:

> . . . the line between speech and action had become blurred and shaky. Embodied cognition, the interdependence of emotion and cognition, the materiality of words and sentences, the transpersonality of mind and subjectivities, the study of intentionality and theory of mind as an outcome of early dyadic life—all these new domains of work and research move us far beyond old dichotomies. The focus on speech as action, on the embodiment and intersubjectivity of speaking and listening, is at the heart of relational ideas.
>
> (p. 15)

Bacal

Finally, Bacal (1998; Bacal & Carlton 2011), a theorist identified mainly with contemporary self psychology, has been developing a therapeutic philosophy, which, similar to the Relational theorists—Ehrenberg, Hoffman, Aron, and Harris—explicitly incorporates both understanding through empathy and relational responsiveness as a functional unity—but with a different theoretical and clinical style.

Bacal's concepts of "optimal responsiveness" (1998) and therapeutic "specificity" (2011) are along similar lines to my thinking about needed relationships and Sander's idea of progressive fittedness.[4] He situates his model in the tradition of Kohut's (1984) two-phase conception of therapeutic action: the first phase emphasizing the achievement of *understanding through empathic immersion*; the second emphasizing *explanation* (mostly of the developmental, "genetic" reasons for a patient's adaptation, and selfobject needs), *through verbal interpretation.* As noted in my earlier review of Kohut's thinking, this had been Kohut's party line throughout most of his career and writing, allowing him to continue to identify with traditional analysis. But Bacal's personal experience as Kohut's analysand told a different story: He found Kohut much more relationally responsive than his theory of technique acknowledged, and this made all the difference for Bacal. It also led to his modifying Kohut's two-step model such that the first step remained understanding through empathic inquiry and attunement, but in the second phase, verbal explanation (based on that understanding) is replaced with "optimal responsiveness"— responding to the patient in whatever unique ways meet each patient's specific therapeutic needs, as expressed and addressed within the specific dynamics, qualities, and constraints of each two-person analytic relationship. In Bacal's words:

> [The] sine qua non of psychoanalytic therapy is not empathy culminated by verbal interpretation . . . , but the entire process that includes understanding the complex mental states of another, and discerning the needed theraperutic response that may or may not be possible within the ineluctably reciprocal process of that particular dyad.
>
> (2011, p. 55)

Bacal's books are replete with examples of his empathic and creative processes as he works toward responding to the, often complex and challenging, needs of his patients, coming up with solutions that are fitted to his patients in much the way I am advocating in this book.

The center will not hold: explicit vs. implicit relational knowing

Even as theorists like Ehrenberg, Hoffman, Aron, Harris, and Bacal have been strongly voicing a more integrative and/or dialectical approach, for the past decade and a half an increasingly influential trend in relational theory has pulled the thinking of many, regarding the relationship between analytic understanding and relational engagement, "to the left." An expanding group of theorists, influenced by infancy and attachment research, and cognitive neuroscience, has been emphasizing implicit (i.e., non-conscious, non-verbal), "procedural," relational factors *over* explicit, symbolically rendered, understanding as the primary curative agent in analytic therapy (e.g., D.N. Stern et al., 1998; Lyons-Ruth et al., 1998; Lyons-Ruth, 1999; Boston Change Process Study Group, 2008, 2010; Schore, 2011; Beebe & Lachman, 2014). Grounding their arguments in findings from cognitive psychology indicating that there are two "distinct and dissociable" memory systems—one for explicit or conscious memory ("knowing that") and the other for non-conscious, implicit or procedural memory ("knowing how") (Lyons-Ruth, 1999)—this group of theorists asserts that, while both learning systems are involved in psychoanalytic interaction and change, the implicit system of intersubjective procedural communication, learning, and knowing, which has its roots in the earliest interactions between mothers and babies, tends to lead, while the explicit system of verbal symbolization tends to follow. Moreover, the implicit system is thought to be more pervasive and thus where most of the therapeutic action takes place. In different language, the emphasis in this line of thought is placed on "right brain to right brain" *as opposed to* "left brain to left brain" communication (Schore, 2011).

Because of the widening influence of this trend in relational/intersubjective theory, I feel it is necessary to examine its underlying assumptions more closely as part of the process of working through toward the more integrated, holistic model implied in the meta-theory of needed relationships. I will refer to this theoretical movement as "IRK theory" or "IRK movement"—an acronym for the term "implicit relational knowing" introduced by Lyons-Ruth et al. (1998) and the Boston Change Process Study Group (D.N. Stern et al., 1998).

The IRK theorists have, in my view, made a major, paradigm changing, contribution by illuminating the nature, scope, and importance of the implicit relational dimension of the analytic exchange, and in so doing have also made a compelling case for greater openness on the part of the analytic community to the explosion of relevant knowledge in the neighboring fields they have drawn from. I will argue, however, that they have framed the issues wrongly by separating implicit engagement from reflective understanding in their therapeutic scheme, especially with respect to therapy with adults, and by privileging the former over the latter (see also S. Stern, 2008). Even though their thinking in some ways extends a trend that was already occurring in relational theory (for example, in the focus on enactments), and even though they frequently cite leading Relationalists in their writings, because their model loses touch with the generative tension in contemporary theory between understanding and engagement, their thinking loses analytic generality and power. To give the reader a beginning sense of the basis for this challenge, and to take us more deeply into the issues involved in trying to clarify the relationship between engagement and understanding, I offer the following brief clinical vignette.

A 50-year-old patient, Mary, faithfully returns with her husband every year to share Thanksgiving with her family of origin, which at this point includes her mother, her sister, and her sister's family. During the five years we had been working together, she had returned from these visits more or less undone by the all-too-familiar pattern of judgmental scrutiny, criticism, negation, and guilt-induction that she encountered at the hands of her mother (and sometimes her sister), and against which she had remained defenseless despite the slow gains she was making in her analysis. In previous years she had literally spent months anxiously anticipating and trying to gird herself for her visits, and months following the visits working with me to restore her shattered sense of self and goodness. While I have what I consider to be a fairly complex theoretical understanding of the nature of Mary's struggle (S. Stern, 2002a, 2002b, 2015, In preparation), and specifically what happened to her when she went home, on the eve of her departure in our fifth year, seemingly unbidden, the thought occurred to me and I said, "Why don't you think of your family members as like the raptors in *Jurassic Park.* You *have* to keep them locked in their cages!" She laughed out loud at this image, but the surprising outcome was that it worked! She came back essentially unscathed, crediting my "advice" for her progress. Moreover, the change held up over time: Her subsequent trips home have not been quite the ordeal they once were.

Prior to this intervention, Mary and I had been immersed in her struggle with her introjected and real family members for years. The imagery that increasingly had been coloring our dialogue around this struggle—imagery from her vivid dream life and my interpretive elaboration of these dream elements—was that of terrible destructiveness and primitive zero-sum games in which one person's survival meant another's psychic murder. The mother had emerged in fantasy images as a ravenous, flesh-eating creature; thus my language came from, and spoke to, Mary's unconscious experience and creativity. She and I had already lived through a lot together, including a prolonged enactment in the second year of our work in which the viability of the treatment had been called into question. (See Chapter 7 for a detailed account of this impasse.) For several years prior to this Thanksgiving intervention, humor and verbal playfulness had come increasingly into our dialogue, delighting us both, and providing what felt to both of us to be a potent affective antidote ("up-regulation") to the quicksand-like nature of Mary's deeply entrenched habits of self-negation and self-excoriation. My quip about keeping the raptors in their cages was a somewhat more forceful and directed expression of the unique form of gallows humor she and I had been co-creating for a while.

This verbal playfulness had become an important resource in our relationship that I/we could draw upon at the point I made my comment. Mary's receptivity to my quip, and her ability to hold and use it when visiting her family, were, of course, inseparable from her experience of me as a very particular new object, which she had slowly begun to internalize over years of work together.

How might an informed analyst, an analyst well versed in the past 60 years of analytic thought about needed relationships, parse the relative contributions of relational engagement and the communication of understanding in my two-sentence intervention? It would, I submit, be an impossible exercise. It would be impossible because, in every word that I spoke, understanding and engagement were inextricably *fused* in an interpenetrating, mutually constituting "mix-up," to borrow loosely from Balint (1968). My intervention was part of a dialogue that embodied a non-linear coalescence of *both* Mary's and my evolving understanding of her struggles *and* our evolving relational engagement (conscious and implicit) in the service of trying to help her with those struggles. The relationship between understanding and engagement in this intervention was not the parallel one described by the Boston Study Group in which the symbolic dimension is separate from and lags behind its older, faster sister, the implicit dimension. If anything, symbolization was the leading element. Rather, the relationship between understanding and engagement exemplified in this vignette was, as Ehrenberg described it over two decades ago, and Aron captures in the quote that begins this chapter, one of complete interpenetration—the two dimensions were seamlessly interwoven and mutually constituting. This is so, I would argue, much of the time in every analysis, even in many moments when the analyst's participation is non-verbal.

Three sources of confusion and murkiness have surrounded this issue: (1) a conflation between what the therapist explicitly says or interprets and her *total understanding and all that she or he implicitly communicates because of that understanding*; (2) a conflation between the patient's *conscious awareness and registration* of what is occurring and being taken in from a given interaction, and *all* of the elements that are actually contained and transmitted in that interaction; and (3) generalizations from mother-infant interaction studies to the realm of adult psychotherapy that do not have the same observational, scientific grounding as the studies themselves or inferences regarding child development, and therefore may be wrongly formulated.

The analyst's total understanding

The point I wish to make here is that, however one positions the verbal/symbolic vs. the implicit relational dimensions in characterizing the analyst's *interventions* or the *observable therapeutic interaction*, the analyst's commitment to seeking an ever-better understanding of the patient and the unfolding process is (or should be) constant and central to everything the analyst does with a patient, whether verbal or non-verbal, interpretive or enactive (in an intentional, positive sense). A corollary of this premise is that, even though our theories may lead us to conclude that *the patient's* verbally symbolized insight or self-understanding is not always necessary for, or central to, analytic growth and transformation, the same does not apply to the analyst's analyzing subjectivity. The patient implicitly relies on the analyst's dedication to reaching ever-better, fuller understandings of him in the context of the analytic relationship and process. A second, related corollary is that, even though we now understand that the analyst's evolving understanding is inseparable from the relational processes within which that understanding emerges, and even though the analyst may arrive at implicit senses or "knowings" regarding how to *be* with a patient at a given point in time without these knowings being fully, consciously symbolized in language, these implicit processes can only occur in an overall context or field in which the analyst is always, ultimately *seeking* the most inclusive understanding possible, both at implicit/intuitive and explicit/symbolic levels. This therapeutic reality should be evident from the fact that every psychoanalytic text written about the nature and centrality of implicit relational processes is written to enhance analysts' *understanding* of such processes, presumably on the premise that such understanding will broaden and enrich analysts' capacities to understand and apprehend what is occurring at that level, and thereby better respond to their patients' total process and needs. Thus, whatever the therapeutic yield of seemingly independent, implicit, not-fully-symbolized, relational processes as they occur in certain analytic interactions, there is no such isolation of implicit processes in the analyst's analyzing subjectivity (except perhaps in a momentary sense): Relational engagement and progressive understanding are always interdependent, interpenetrating, and co-evolving in the analyst's total participation, and thus "saturate" all that is occurring in the interaction.

It is helpful here to consider the differences between the patient's and the analyst's subjectivities, given their different roles in the therapeutic relationship. Terms such as "intersubjective system," "two-person psychology," and "mutual regulation" emphasize the *similarities* between the patient and therapist: Both are human beings engaged in a system involving mutual influence and regulation. But they fail to capture the equally important reality that the analyst's subjectivity-as-analyst is far more complex than the patient's subjectivity-as-patient. The analyst's subjectivity, *including her embodied subjectivity*, contains all that the analyst has learned (through both scholarship and experience) in the service of performing the transformational functions (Bion, 1965; Bollas, 1987) involved in analytic work. These transformational functions require complex conscious and unconscious *processing and relational capacities* that reflect both the myriad analytic frames of reference learned and internalized by the analyst through scholarly immersion in analytic (and related) ideas, and the more implicit forms of understanding gleaned from clinical analytic experience (and, of course, life experience). These two forms of understanding are hardly separate or "dissociable," but rather inform each other, are integrated in infinitely complex ways, and are expressed not only in the content of what the analyst says but in her total presence, voice, and implicit communications of all kinds at all times (see also S. Stern, 2008). They constitute what I referred to in Chapter 2 as the analyst's *wisdom.* Understood in this more complex way, the imparting of understanding does not occur only through explicit interpretations but rather through an extremely complex form of the "dyadic expansion of consciousness" (Tronick, 1998, 2007) brought about in interactions that are at all times informed, or at least affected, by the analyst's explicit *and* implicit understanding and her transformational capacities.

Part of the murkiness here results from the fact that the theorists who emphasize the bifurcation of explicit and implicit processing (for example, D.N. Stern et al., 1998, in their seminal paper on " . . . the something more than interpretation") are still using the classical Freudian model of interpretation-leading-to-insight as their prototype of explicit, symbolized knowing and communication. In that model explicit, discreet verbal formulations of the patient's intrapsychic dynamic structure and process, delivered by a detached, neutral analyst, were seen as the vehicle of transformation.

This stereotype does not take into account the dramatic revisions in the model of the analyst's reflective activity that have occurred in the past 60 years. Bion (1962, 1970) stands out as offering a different model in which the analyst's internal processing of implicit emotional experience, much like the digestive processes of the human body, leads to transformations of raw (implicit) experience into more "contained," metabolized, symbolizable experience, which can then serve as a basis for transformative interaction with the patient. That transformational exchange might or might not take the form of explicit interpretation. Most importantly and tellingly, the analyst's capacity to process emotional experience in this way is potentially *freeing* to both parties—freeing in the sense of an enhanced capacity for generative processing through dreams, reveries, memories, fantasies, associations (including somatic "associations"), *thinking* in general, and *dialogue* (Symington, 1983; Ogden, 1994, 1997, 2005; Eigen, 1996; S. Stern, 2009c). In other words, the yield of the analyst's processing capacities, conscious and unconscious, is not so much the communication of discreet understandings as the freeing up of the patient's own processing capacities in order to be able to think and speak about, and thus grow from, their emotional experience.

I am focusing on Bion's "theory of thinking" since it offers the most systematic revision of the Freudian model of the analyst's cognitive processing and interpretive activity. However, other models, for example Loewald's (1979) more informal, evocative theoretical formulation of the analytic process, move in a similar direction:

> It seems to me that an interpretation is not so much the result of understanding as it is the means by which understanding proceeds. This has to do with the intimate interrelations between thought and language . . . Understanding as an act . . . is impossible unless the patient lends himself and is open to our understanding . . . unless the patient feels understood we feel that we have not fully understood him. *Understanding would seem to be an act that involves some sort of mutual engagement, a particular form of the meeting of minds.*
>
> (pp. 381–382, emphasis added)

Elsewhere, Loewald (1960), sounding very much like Bion, characterizes psychic health as the capacity to integrate (move back and forth between) the unconscious and preconscious registers of experience. Interpretations, to be effective, must emanate from this capacity in the analyst and aim to develop the same capacity in the patient: "Language, in its most specific function in analysis, as interpretation, is thus a creative act similar to that in poetry, where language is found for phenomena, contexts, connections, experiences not previously known and speakable . . . " (1960, p. 242).

Ogden (1997), nearly four decades later, with the benefit of both Bion's and Loewald's perspectives, echoes Loewald: "In attempting to capture something of the experience of being alive in words, the words themselves must be alive. Words, when they are living and breathing, are like musical chords" (p. 4).

Explicit and implicit processes in the patient's subjectivity-as-patient

Although the analyst's subjective participation is more complex than the patient's, the bifurcation of implicit and explicit processing also oversimplifies the patient's subjectivity, especially as an analytic treatment progresses. As I have argued previously:

> Like the Boston Study Group, I view the analyst's verbal-symbolic communication as emerging *from* IRK [implicit relational knowing], but think one of its primary functions is the transformation *of* IRK, including transformation of the ways the patient implicitly relates to himself or herself. Once the analyst's verbal and interpretive statements have served this transformational function (which may occur in one dramatic interchange or require repetition of certain themes over years) . . . they are "reabsorbed" back into IRK (IRK contains "residues" of verbal-symbolic dialogue). This may explain why former patients often do not remember specific interpretations. It is not that the interpretations were not significant; it is that their impact is "remembered" at the implicit relational level.
>
> (S. Stern, 2008, pp. 505–506)

Once a good-enough analytic treatment is underway the patient's subjectivity becomes progressively transformed by all that has occurred intersubjectively, and contains or embodies both the residues of previous analytic understandings and newly acquired processing and reflective capacities that the patient is developing in the context of the analytic work. Non-linear dynamic systems theorists such as Coburn (2014) and Marks-Tarlow (2008) have been especially clear about this cumulative complexity.

Taking my "raptor" intervention as a case in point, it was my (implicit) hope, of course, that the particular fusion of implicit and explicit messages contained in my metaphorical quip *would* impact Mary's implicit functioning when visiting her family. And indeed, that is what seems to have happened: The subjective residue of our total interchange seemed implicitly to calm and guide her through the treacherous waters of her 3-day holiday visit. Moreover, the same residues, probably in combination with the increased sense of mastery following this more successful visit, continued to help her in subsequent visits. Again, I ask: How could one possibly separate the workings of implicit and explicit knowing in Mary's improved functioning with her family? We don't necessarily want our patients to remember everything we have said; we want their total functioning (implicit and explicit) to have been transformed by all that has occurred in the analysis.

Another source of confusion and murkiness is the changing understanding of what it is that the analyst (and patient) most *need to understand*. Insight and understanding are no longer exclusively about the patient's intrapsychic experience, conflicts, anxieties, defenses, and desires taken in isolation; they have expanded to include the bi-directional interaction between relational experience and self-experience as it emerges and comes into focus in the analytic relationship, the patient's outside relationships, dreams, and in associations of all kinds—especially to memories of the patient's early relationships. Through these progressive glimpses and symbolized "capturings" of the patient's experiential world, analyst and patient gradually co-construct a "moving picture" of the patient's experience of self-in-relation-to-others. The analyst approaches this interpretive project with a plethora of models held loosely in the background regarding how different kinds of relational experience affect self-experience and capacities of all kinds, and of how different kinds of self-experience may affect intersubjective interaction. For example, my general understanding of such matters tells me that ultimately Mary will need to grieve the loss of what she never received from her family in order to more fully separate from them internally, but that in order to tolerate this grieving process, she will need to feel connected enough to me as a new object who *both* understands her *and* is relationally invested in her in a caring, reliable way (S. Stern, In preparation).

My Thanksgiving intervention implicitly incorporated this understanding as a background factor. The evocation of the raptor image and the ironic injunction to keep her family members "locked in their cages" captured (implicitly interpreted) the dual reality that (a) at the interpersonal level, her family members actually still behave in destructive (anger and fear-provoking) ways, while (b) at the intrapsychic level, it is Mary who now, at age 50, gives them too much power due to their archaic object status; and it is she who, ultimately, must actualize her potential capacity to take back this power into herself. At the same time, the contextualization of these implied insights within the affectionate, spontaneous, humorous, and supportive qualities of our exchange performatively conveyed the recognition that her felt connection to me as a new object is essential in order for her to *use* these insights as I intended them—that is, to embolden her to contemplate separating from her family members in the ways she needs to. Further, to underline the complexity of the interpenetration of the explicit and the implicit, the tone and implicit "atmosphere" of my quip was not one of exhortation, reflecting an over-focus on Mary's "symptom" or a need on my part to get her to change (Ogden & Gabbard, 2010); but rather one of play and irony, reflecting both my understanding of Mary's susceptibility to feeling criticized and deficient if expected to do something of which she feels incapable, and my respect for the fact that change of this sort can only occur under Mary's own initiative (or, in Winnicott's [1960a, 1969] language, within her "sphere of omnipotence"). In such ways, I would argue, engagement both reflects *and* affects understanding, and understanding shapes and influences the moment-to-moment, thoughtfully spontaneous, improvisational generation of ever-changing forms of engagement. How can they be separated? Who would want to?

Extrapolations from infant research to adult treatment

One of the lures, and rhetorical strategies, of the proliferating IRK literature applying principles gleaned from mother-infant observation studies to adult treatment is the implication that they are more scientifically based because the principles are derived from empirical research. I would argue that, while the principles and theories emanating from infancy research have profoundly changed and enriched our understanding of infant and child development, and certain aspects of human nature and learning more generally, their applicability to the adult treatment context needs to be carefully considered. Any comprehensive attempt at such an examination is beyond the scope and purposes of this book. Here, I will only pose the question whether the various generalizations being made have the same levels of "inferential validity" (i.e., are equally logical and compelling). Of the three major generalizations made or implied in this literature, only one seems to me virtually inarguable, while the other two seem at best questionable, and, in my view, are probably wrong (D.N. Stern et al., 1998; Boston Change Process Study Group, 2008, 2010).

The first, more credible inference is that, just as implicit (unsymbolized or not-fully-verbally-symbolized) relational processes are central in infant-mother interactions, they are also central or at least pervasive in the communication processes of adult treatment. Here I believe the, now extensive, literature on the "something more than interpretation" (D.N. Stern et al., 1998) has been and continues to be enormously illuminating and clinically compelling. The recognition that much of what is happening in the clinical exchange is occurring out of conscious, linguistically symbolized awareness, including forms of "micro-interaction" that are both too brief and moving too quickly to be consciously registered or controlled (Beebe & Lachmann, 2014), seems both humbling and potentially empowering. It is humbling to realize, once again, that our conscious, intentional subjectivities are but a part (probably the lesser part) of our total "going on being" (Winnicott, 1960a), and that our subjective experience at all levels (conscious, unconscious, embodied, fantasized) is embedded in social ecosystems (including therapeutic dyads) that shape and control us outside of our awareness. It is potentially empowering in that such awareness potentially expands our capacities for attunement to our patients at levels not previously consciously perceived, and expands our repertoires of response potentials to include non-verbal and procedural forms of participation and improvisation. These gains in understanding, attunement, and clinical range are well illustrated in the clinical examples adduced in this literature to demonstrate the operation of implicit processes in adult therapeutic interaction and transformation (e.g., D.N. Stern et al., 1998; Beebe, 2004;

Beebe & Lachmann, 2014; Lyons-Ruth et al., 1998; Knoblauch, 2000). From the standpoint of the meta-theory of needed relationships and progressive fittedness advocated in this book, this extrapolation from infancy research regarding the pervasiveness and nature of implicit, procedural processes in adult analytic treatment would seem only to advance our capacities to achieve such fittedness with a wider range of patients.

The second and third major generalizations are more problematic. These have been asserted in a two-fold contention, first advanced by the Boston Study Group (D.N. Stern et al., 1998), that: (a) the implicit, non-verbal forms of communication observed in mother-infant interaction studies represent a *distinct dimension of interaction*, which, in adult psychotherapy, is separable from a different dimension—i.e., cognitive, symbolized, linguistic communication, the prototype for which is the classical therapeutic model of interpretation leading to insight; and (b) interaction in the implicit realm is *more centrally involved in analytic transformation* than verbal interpretation in the explicit realm. None of the authors at the forefront of the IRK theoretical movement deny that interpretation, and verbal (i.e., symbolized) communication more generally, still constitute an important dimension of analytic interaction and the change process. But, they tend to view it as distinct from, slower than, and when it gets down to it, secondary to, what is occurring at the non-verbal, implicit relational level. I have already given most of my arguments against these assertions earlier in the chapter. Here, I will add one further argument that has to do with *the logic* of how these theorists are extrapolating from mother-infant interaction research to the adult treatment context. To aid in this argument I begin by quoting in full a description of a 20-second interaction between a mother and 4-month-old offered by Beebe and Lachmann (2014) as an example of "disruption and repair" in a mother-infant pair who, the authors know, are on their way to establishing a secure attachment relationship (as assessed at 12 months). I should say that the following is the authors' summarized narrative of the sequence rather than the second-by-second microanalysis, which they also provide.

> The film begins with the mother and infant looking at each other. The mother says a drawn-out "Hiii" as she leans in and smiles widely. The infant vocalizes with a slightly positive tone and smiles. His hands play with the blanket on the seat as his head moves a bit forward, while

> he continues to look at mother. Mother repeats "Hiii" while moving in closer to the infant with a partial "loom," and she laughs. ("Loom" movements are ones in which the mother's head and face move in very close to the infant's face, within a few inches.) The infant quickly becomes distressed, frowns, and moves his head back as he raises his arms. He seems to have reacted to the loom. He looks away from his mother and whimpers. The mother immediately moves back into an upright position and sobers.
>
> The mother offers her hands to the infant, "Here, take my hands," with a lilting prosody. The infant takes her fingers, while the mother sings, "That's my fingers." The infant's eyes follow the mother's hand movements until she begins to raise his hands. The infant then looks at his mother. Mother smiles and sings in rhythm with the movements of their hands while the infant gazes at her, with a slight positive expression.
>
> The mother moves her hands down onto the infant's lap, and the infant still holds on to his mother's fingers. The mother now has a broad, highly positive smile. The infant smiles too, almost as broadly as his mother. The mother's smile slightly decreases as she says, "Can you say "ahhh," as she slowly leans in close to the infant, another partial loom. The infant giggles and lowers his head, and then moves his head back up, meanwhile continuing to gaze at his mother. Both infant and mother match the rhythm of their mouth and head movements.
>
> (2014, p. 12)

The first point I want to make about this remarkably precise and alive rendering of what is apparently a very telling interaction sequence (in regard to the health of this dyad), is that what we are "seeing" here is not a dimension of the interaction between mother and baby; it is the total interaction of two whole persons using their entire mind/brains to engage each other in a complex interaction that seems to be mostly about connecting, attuning, enjoying, playing, repairing missteps, and, in two brief moments, teaching language. What stands out to me is that the mother is energetically, even passionately, using her whole self to attune to and play with the child as he is now, in each present moment. While it is true, the infant does not yet have language, the mother attempts to connect with her child using the non-verbal "language" or "languages" he currently does possess, and, in fact, embeds some language instruction in her play: e.g., "That's my fingers"; "Can you say "ahhh?" Thus, part of what is going on implicitly (actually, it's pretty explicit!) is that the mother is "pulling" the infant toward symbolization and linguistic communication with a conscious intention to do so.

My second point follows from the first: To extrapolate from this vignette that the most important "dimension" of adult therapeutic interaction is what is going on at the non-verbal, mostly non-conscious, implicit, procedural level seems illogical and "unfair" to both the mother-infant and therapist-patient dyads. It seems to me the more logical, accurate, and useful extrapolation is from the mother-infant interaction to the *total interaction* between adult patients and therapists. Just as the mother is using her entire mind/brain/body to grasp and communicate with the infant's total mind/brain/body within the frame (set up by the investigators) of engaging in enjoyable, playful interaction, so do therapists, within their frame, seek to use *their* entire mind/brain/bodies to communicate with their patients' total mind/brain/bodies in the service of their task of helping patients analytically (and relationally) with their struggles.

I would argue further that, in the clinical context at least, the therapist's efforts to understand or cognitively grasp a patient's psychic reality is not a separate or separable "dimension" of the clinical task. Rather, *all* of the ways that an analyst is processing and communicating with the patient, including all uses of language, are, in the clinical context, *procedural,* and are *emergent* from the analyst's implicit processing of the total interaction on an ongoing basis. (Harris, 2009, pp. 15–16, citing Bahktin [1981] and Lakoff and Johnson [1980, 1999], makes essentially this same point.) That is, everything the therapist says and does, *including* everything within her awareness and therapeutic intention, is occurring in the context of the overall, mostly implicit *procedure* of seeking and achieving progressive fittedness in the service of helping the patient. In this context, as I argued earlier in the chapter, all efforts to understand, all the processes through which understanding emerges, and all choices about what understanding to communicate to a patient at a given moment and how best to do that, are of a piece with and in the service of the total therapeutic procedure, and are inseparable from all that is happening relationally, emotionally, and unconsciously (or non-consciously). Thus, rather than thinking of interpretations as operating at a different, less immediate and powerful level of exchange, it seems to me that, as with the mother and infant in Beebe and Lachmann's vignette, therapists should think in terms of using their whole mind/brain/bodies (as a complex system) to engage the whole mind/brain/bodies of their patients, including all of the "languages" or registers through which their patients are trying to engage *them* (the therapists) and make themselves (the patients) known to their therapists. In addition, of course, like the mother in Beebe and Lachmann's study, one of the ways we engage our patients is a kind of implicit instruction: teaching them the symbolic "language" of psychological/emotional/relational experience and communication (Stolorow, 2006), thereby "pulling" them toward greater emotional intelligence and fluency, and making possible what Fonagy and his co-authors describe as the capacity for "mentalization" (Fonagy et al., 2002).

Framed in this way, much of what therapists say to, or do with, patients—for example, what I said to Mary about "keeping the raptors locked in their cages"—does not tend to fall neatly into pre-existing categories of therapist participation. Rather, they are *contoured* to the patient and the present moment, just as the mother in the study contoured her "interventions" to her baby. In this regard I share Ogden's (2009) view that:

> A critically important aspect of . . . psychoanalysis is the creation of ways of talking with each patient that are unique to *that* patient in *that* moment of the analysis. When I speak of talking differently with each patient, I am referring not simply to the unselfconscious use of different tones of voice, rhythms of speech, choice of words, types of formality and informality, and so on, but also to particular ways of being with, and communicating with, another person that could exist between no other two people on this planet.
>
> (p. 2, emphasis in the original)

What makes Sander different?

Both Sander, in his writings touching on adult psychotherapy (e.g., 1995, 2002, 2008), and, by extension, I, in this book, would seem to be making the same kinds of extrapolations from infancy research to adult treatment that I am finding problematic in the IRK theorists' work. Indeed, Sander was a member of the original Boston Study Group, whose 1998 paper launched the IRK theoretical movement (D.N. Stern et al., 1998). In fact, he was obviously an influential member, given the number of his concepts that the group incorporated into their synthesis in that initial paper. I did not know Sander personally; nor do I know about the inner workings of the BCPSG. Thus I don't know how he felt about the ultimate end product of the group's collaboration. What I do know is that Sander's use of his own concepts, and his thinking in general as I understand it, move in the exact opposite direction of where the BCPSG ended up in that paper.

Sander's thinking does not focus on, or attempt to parse, the internal sub-divisions of human interaction, but instead looks at mother and baby (and by extension, patient and therapist) as whole persons coordinating their roles and intentions within a complex human system. Sander's primary interest and concern—indeed, what I sense to have been the generative passion of his life's work—was his quest to understand the mysterious intersubjective processes through which the individual child or patient, in *all* of his diffuse complexity as a living system, self-organizes into states of relative coherence (identity) and develops a sense of personal agency and well-being. Drawing upon the work of biologist Paul Weiss (1970), Sander proposed the principle of "matched specificities" or, in human psychological terms, "specificity in recognition," as a central principle and process through which two people interact in the service of the progressive development, competence, agency, and coherence of one of them. In Sander's (1995) words, the senses of identity and personal agency develop from repeated intersubjective experiences in which the way one "knows" oneself is "matched" by the way one is "known" by the other. Elsewhere Sander wrote: "[Specificity in] recognition can be thought of as a way of representing how one individual comes to *savor the wholeness of another* . . . the critical condition for the reorganization of both interacting partners as they progress toward new integration" (2008, p. 169; emphasis added). Somehow, it seems, these core principles—the essential spirit—of Sander's views on human development and change got lost in the BPCSG's strategy of *isolating and elevating as preeminent* one particular dimension of the change process.

The main "units of analysis" in Sander's model are each individual, the two-person system, and the evolving developmental/therapeutic tasks or aims that the system is organizing itself to help (primarily) one member achieve. The idea of two whole persons (therapist and patient) organizing as a complex system directed toward a highly complex form of problem-solving that is simultaneously intrapsychic and intersubjective for both parties orients us to the fact that both the patient and analyst, as members of such a problem-solving system, are at all times utilizing the totality of their individual and joint problem-solving capacities and all of the mental sub-systems (conscious and unconscious, implicit and explicit, reflective and embodied, left brain and right brain) that are in service to this over-arching organizing purpose.[5] How all of those mental sub-systems are engaged and interact from moment to moment is dictated by whatever emerging proximal form the developmental/problem-solving process is taking in each moment, session, and period of work, governed ultimately by the *principle of necessity*. (See Chapter 4.)

By framing the analytic process in this way I am underlining the *irreducible density* of the analytic dialogue or exchange (see also Coburn, 2014). My two-sentence intervention with Mary was irreducibly dense, representing an emergent "invention" of mine, in the context of our *total* relationship and shared understandings, in the moment when I made it. In Sander's terms, it proved to be a good "match," in that moment, with Mary's current state and her implicit developmental aims and struggles.

Synthesis

To return to the main question of this chapter—the relationship between understanding and relational engagement in psychoanalytic treatment and theory—now, hopefully, disentangled from, but also informed by, the discourse on implicit vs. explicit knowing, I will summarize my own current take on the question. It seems to me that the two currents of thought in contemporary psychoanalysis that I have identified—one pertaining to the progressive illumination of the patient's truth, the aim of which is the patient's increasing capacity to "live from" or in accord with that truth (Ogden & Gabbard, 2010; Symington, 2012), the other pertaining to the optimal forms of relational engagement for bringing about transformations in the patient's ways of being, relating, and experiencing in directions the patient implicitly wishes to move—come together under the rubric of Sander's ideas of specificity of recognition and fittedness, and my meta-theory of needed relationships. That is, the analyst is *at all times* seeking *both* to expand and deepen her *understanding* of the patient and what is occurring interactively in the analytic field, *and* to *engage* the patient in ways that are optimally and uniquely conducive to the patient's growth and transformation as these transformational aims are progressively revealed, and evolve, over the course of treatment (Ehrenberg, 1992). Seen in this way, it becomes clear that the analyst is never "off the hook" (Hoffman, 1998) of seeking simultaneously to achieve maximal understanding *and* optimal engagement, and thus, as Ehrenberg was the first to articulate, to *combine* them in ways that best advance the analytic process in the moment.

Moreover, in this framework it is recognized that the analyst's understanding and forms of relational engagement are mutually constituting dimensions of the intersubjective analytic experience and change process (Aron, 2012). The analyst's complex understanding of the elements at play in the analytic process infuses and shapes her implicit experience and ways of being an analyst at all times. Further, the analyst's current level or quality of understanding, including her moment-to-moment relationship to her own internal experience, even if not explicitly formulated or voiced, exerts an implicit influence on the patient's current experience—his experience of the analyst, the analytic process, and himself (Symington, 1983; Davies, 2004[6]). Conversely, the quality of relational engagement, moment to moment, exerts enormous shaping influence: on the quality of the patient's participation, including his unfolding capacities to reflect on, feel, and speak his previously unthinkable emotional experience; on what both parties are able to "hear," "see," and sense within the field; and on how that data is processed, formulated, creatively elaborated, and communicated. (Principle [Principle]s 4 and 9 of Needed Relationships—See Introduction.) In short, the synergistic combination of understanding and engagement creates an *intersubjective medium* through which the mysterious, transformational alchemy of analysis—the cumulative "dyadic expansion of consciousness" (Tronick, 1998, 2007)—takes place.

To distill the ideas developed in this chapter down to their abstract essence, I borrow from, and take the liberty of adding to, Bion's (e.g., 1962, 1970) famous symbols. In the ceaseless flow of interaction between patient and analytic therapist there is always the intention and effort on the analyst's part to understand, and the current yield of that effort—Bion's "**K**." But there is also the constant flow of relational engagement (Ehrenberg, 1992; Grossmark, 2012a) and the analyst's constant effort to find ways of engaging that are optimally productive or connecting, which I will call "**R**." I think of the total flow of **K** and **R** as emergent from Bion's "**O**" (the ultimate, total, implicit, mysterious, largely unknowable reality of the patient, the analyst, and their interaction within the analytic field). Following Bion (1970), the optimal attitude for the apprehension of **O** is a radical openness signified by his injunction to approach the session "without memory or desire." I think of this state as an open, creative, intuitive receptivity and surrender to the process; and in an analytic couple working well together, this can at times become a *co*-creative *co*-receptivity and *mutual* surrender at the implicit level. Bion believed that this radical openness to the psychic realities which lie beyond current understanding, combined with a necessary capacity for tolerating ambiguity, confusion, and uncertainty, sometimes for extended periods, has the best chance of yielding an "evolution" from the experience and apprehension of **O** to new, emergent (though always incomplete) understandings: $\mathbf{O} \longrightarrow \mathbf{K}$. What I am adding is that the effort to "enter" and apprehend the **O** of the interaction also leads to *emergent evolutions in **R***—the evolving forms of relational engagement within which **K** is embedded and communicated, but which also are, to some degree, shaped and framed *by* **K**. Thus I would modify Bion's formulation to: $\mathbf{O} \longrightarrow \mathbf{RK}$, where **RK** represents the evolving, interpenetrating, mutually constituting, multiplicative relationship between understanding and relational engagement. By "multiplicative" I invoke Ehrenberg's (1992, p. 67) idea that "the integration of the affective and the analytic gives each more scope." These evolutions in **RK** generate transformations "**(*T*)**" in the **O** of the total ongoing interaction and mental states of both parties—transformations that we hope are productive but are always complex, emergent, and unpredictable. We then, ongoingly, turn our attention, our "analytic instrument," our creative receptivity, curiosity, and relational "readiness," to the now-transformed **O**, which in turn yields new evolutions in **RK**. Thus, the analytic process over time could be represented as: $\mathbf{O}_1 \longrightarrow \mathbf{R}_1\mathbf{K}_1 \longrightarrow (T) \longrightarrow \mathbf{O}_2 \longrightarrow \mathbf{R}_2\mathbf{K}_2 \longrightarrow (T) \longrightarrow \ldots\ldots \mathbf{O}_\infty \longrightarrow \mathbf{R}_\infty\mathbf{K}_\infty$

This symbolic account requires one further clarification of the meaning of **R**. The analyst's moment-to-moment relational engagement, we know, is complex and tricky because there are always at least two general aspects to it: the forms of relating that fall within our more-or-less conscious therapeutic intentionality, and our total relational engagement of the moment, which always includes unconscious, unintentional, enactive elements. Indeed, these elements have become, in our post-Bionian era, an important component of **O**—i.e., an important part of the total inter-psychic reality of the session that we are seeking to apprehend, understand, and transform. The relationship between these two relational dimensions is extremely, really impossibly, complex. For the purposes of the synthesis I am trying to represent here with these symbols, **R** is being used to refer primarily to the first aspect: those elements of the analyst's relational engagement that fall within her therapeutic intentionality (both conscious and implicit). The second aspect—the unintentional, unconscious, enactive elements of the analyst's relational participation—are, in this symbolic synthesis, considered part of **O**. This is appropriate because, even as the unconscious aspect may be pervasively present, my interest in this chapter mainly concerns the forms of relational engagement that are part of the analyst's therapeutic intentionality, very broadly construed.

Though admittedly experience-distant, and thus perhaps off-putting to some readers, I find this symbolic distillation helpful because it captures the essence of the holistic sensibility intended in the meta-theory of needed relationships, and, I believe, in Sander's theory of specificity of recognition and connection. Rather than approaching the analytic process armed with theoretical categories—categories of patient participation (implicit vs. explicit; emotional vs. cognitive/reflective; etc.) or therapist participation (non-verbal, interpretive, empathic, self-expressive, containing, etc.)—the abstractness of **RK** orients the analyst away from theory toward: (a) the unique and ever-changing complexity of each patient and dyad from session to session and moment to moment; (b) the importance of seeking to apprehend the uniqueness of what is happening in every session, moment to moment (Ogden, 1999; Peltz, 2012); and (c) the uniquely improvised amalgam of communicated (and uncommunicated) understanding, and expressed (and unexpressed) relational/emotional "with-ness," that constitute the therapist's live effort to meet what is happening in a way that causes the patient to feel met, known and helped. This is not to say that we don't need our theories. How we understand **RK** at any given moment is always, necessarily, theory saturated; without our theories **RK** would be an empty, useless term. But my intention, similar, I believe, to Bion's

(1970), and more recently Ogden's (2009), is to place the irreducibly unique patient, and the unfolding analytic process, which is unlike any other, above theory in the live moment that we encounter them, such that our total response in a given moment or session is a unique amalgam of **RK**, inspired by, and fitted to, the "need of the moment."

An ordinary clinical example

At a certain point I became aware that, in my work with Hillary, an accomplished, successfully married, but obsessively anxious woman in her late 40s whom I had been seeing for about 6 months, I was offering a lot of helpful advice and "wisdom" regarding how to deal with her adult children and her family-of-origin members, all of whom caused her great "stress" and worry in different ways. With her children this often took the form of worry, after the fact, about things she had done or said with them by way of offering concern or guidance. Once I noticed what *I* was doing, *I* began to worry about this myself, in a non-specific way (Why am I talking so much? Why am I engaging with Hillary in this particular way?), so decided to say out loud that I noticed myself doing that more than is usual for me, and wondered why. She was surprised by my odd question because we hadn't previously done much talking about our relationship. But she was also intrigued.

We both agreed that the things I said in the service of enlightening her usually felt pertinent and were helping her both to gain understanding and to reposition herself in various ways in her familial relationships. From that point on, however, I tried to be more aware of what I was doing. It wasn't long before I saw, and shared with her, the parallel between my experience with her and her feeling of over-involvement with her children in the sense of offering protective/supportive guidance and then worrying about having done so. I also made a link between these patterns and *the lack* of any helpful guidance received from her parents as a child. Hillary's father was kind but self-absorbed, hypochondriacal, and preoccupied with his business, while her mother was highly critical and controlling, frequently traumatizing Hillary with unpredictable, rageful attacks for failing to conform to her (the mother's) moment-to-moment, often unstated, expectations. "How could you do this to me?" was the mother's angry refrain. Interestingly, during this period in our work, one of Hillary's adult (college age) children had a dream that his mother was in danger, and he was trying to warn and protect *her*—a dream that made Hillary worry about why he felt a need to protect her!

At this point a shift began to occur in our interactions—a move in the direction of "staying with" Hillary's states of worry and tension as opposed to the more active mode of "helping her gain perspective" that I/we had been in. It became clear that she was in a more or less constant state of tension or worry about one thing or another. She associated to her mother growing up—her intrusive, unstoppable rages. All Hillary could do was hide in the closet. I labeled her mother's unpredictable rages a childhood trauma, and Hillary's constant anxiety a form of PTSD. She wondered how we should "approach" the problem, how she would "work it through." I said we would have to look to her, follow her lead.

In the next session she began by saying: "This is like Yoga class: I have to work hard to stop my swirling mind in order to focus on what's happening internally." I asked: "But what is the quality of your swirling mind?" Both of our thoughts again went to her childhood. I said I imagined a child living in a constant state of vigilance, fear, and pain. She recalled using reading as an escape—from her world and into other worlds. She associated to the book she was reading in her women's reading group—David Foster Wallace's *Infinite Jest.* She described Wallace as "brilliant and tortured" and the book as creating "a swirling chaotic world." I wrote down after the session that I "relaxed and was quieter as I simply took an interest in her mind and how it works."

Several sessions later, after a two-week break, Hillary described having, one night, felt panic as she lay in bed unable to get back to sleep. But then, "I thought of your voice, encouraging me to look at what's there and to stay with it. That was comforting, calming, and I got back to sleep." She also reported several situations with family members in which she found herself feeling calmer and "less apologetic" about her actions.

Then, in a subsequent session, I found myself again having the strong impulse to offer her perspective and "wisdom" about struggles she was reporting with her adult children. After telling her I was feeling that impulse again, I went ahead and offered the guidance anyway. She found it quite helpful and grounding. I ended the session saying that I was now aware of a back-and-forth pattern in our sessions between offering guidance and support on the one hand, and simply staying with her anxious states on the other, both of which I assumed were related to her traumatic *dis*regulation, and the help she *didn't* receive with *self*-regulation, as a child.

Discussion

During this early period in my work with Hillary I became aware of an aspect of the **O** (total reality) of my interactions with her—a certain pattern of relating (**R**). By calling attention to it as I did—noticing it out loud without judging it or necessarily trying to do anything about it—I expanded both the **R** and **K** of our interaction to include a new form of engagement—verbal reflection on, and curiosity about, how we had been spontaneously engaging with each other. The result was the beginning of associative links to other relational patterns and experiences in Hillary's childhood and adult life. **R** and **K** were both evolving and interacting, seemingly in synergistic ways, all the while impacting the **O** of Hillary's experience and our relationship. Significantly, one of the ways **R** and **K** interacted here involved the uniquely analytic "relationship" we, at my instigation, were developing with *the process of seeking understanding*. That is, not only was our relationship to each other evolving, so was our relationship to the process of investigation and understanding itself. In this sense, **R** and **K** became even more fused and mutually constituting.

Out of this fusion of **R** and **K** a shift in **R** occurred in the direction of a more standard analytic "staying with" and empathically exploring the sources of Hillary's constant anxiety states. This led to a deepening of **K**, as the traumatic nature of Hillary's childhood experience of her mother came into focus as never before. This, in turn, led to a further shift in **R**: When Hillary asked how she would "work through" her early trauma, I expressed confidence that "following her lead" was the necessary and best approach. This, in turn, led to a further expansion of **K** as we approached her "swirling mind," less with the intention to immediately relieve the swirling than to understand it. This generated memories of her dissociative, self-regulatory use of reading novels as a child. Finally, all of this coalesced in some evidence of Hillary's beginning internalization of both **R** and **K**: As she lay in bed in a panic she could hear my voice encouraging her to "stay with" whatever is there, and this was calming.

This brief period of analytic work, understood as a co-evolution in **R** and **K**, provides a simple example of what I mean by ***contouring*** (see Chapter 3). The co-occurring, evolving transformations in understanding and forms of relational engagement were uniquely and progressively fitted to my, mostly intuitive, implicit, sense of what Hillary and our analytic process "needed" in the service of her mostly implicit aim of mastering her early trauma and resulting chronic anxiety, and, as things evolved, her present-day relationship with her mother. Part of this contouring was a subtle, unplanned rhythm of my "first taking the baton, then handing it back to Hillary" as I alternated between offering helpful guidance and encouraging Hillary to "stay with" whatever she was experiencing and see where her associations took her and us.

Summary

To summarize the major points in this long chapter:

1. The relational paradigm and theoretical movement (broadly construed) has introduced many forms of relational engagement as potential contributors to therapeutic action.
2. With these expanding relational possibilities, the theorized relationship between communicated understanding (so central in traditional psychoanalysis) and relational engagement has become increasingly complex and murky.
3. Some of the major formulations of this issue by prominent relational authors and schools of thought were selectively reviewed and critiqued. Weiss and Sampson, Mitchell, Ehrenberg, Hoffman, Aron, Harris, and Bacal, each in their own way, recognized the inextricability of understanding and relational engagement, which I view as a core principle in the process of achieving progressive fittedness between patient and analyst.
4. I reviewed and critiqued the current trend in relational theory, which (influenced by findings from neighboring scientific fields, especially mother-infant observation studies) privileges the implicit (non-verbal, procedural) relational dimension of analytic interaction over the explicit (verbal, cognitive) dimension.
5. I singled out Sander from other psychoanalytic mother-infant researcher/theorists as adopting a more holistic systems approach that does not parse or privilege one dimension of therapist-patient interaction over another.

6 I presented my own current synthesis, represented by the symbolic formulation: **O ➔ RK ➔ (T) ➔ O . . .**, a modification of Bion's (1970) famous formulation: **O ➔ K ➔ (T) ➔ O.**
7 I offered a brief clinical sequence (which took place over several months) in which there was a progressive contouring of my understanding in tandem with various forms of spontaneously arising relational engagement.

Notes

1 This epigraph is cited with the author's permission.
2 I should note that Orange (1995, 2012), on her own, has fully embraced a philosophy of "emotional availability": responding to patients' relational needs in whatever form seems to fit their need of the moment. She even coined a term—"developmental enactment"—to differentiate these more positive, developmentally supportive engagements from the more problematic kind.
3 For another particularly dramatic and instructive example of this sequence *from* engagement *to* understanding, see Weisel-Barth's (2011) paper, "Katherine: A Long Hard Case." In this 20+ year treatment of a severely traumatized, chaotically organized, depressed, and often un-lucky borderline patient, it was only after decades of Weisel-Barth going way off the traditional analytic map in her protective and ultimately loving responses to Katherine's suicidal crises and seemingly endless needs for everything *but* analytic self-reflection, that Katherine came to a point when *she* finally *wanted*, and explicitly asked for, a more traditional, restrained, analytic dialogue oriented toward self-exploration, reflection and understanding.
4 A detailed comparison of Bacal's model and the one advanced in this book would take us too far afield of the central narrative. Our work is very much in the same spirit, and uses much of the same language. The main differences seem to be in our respective idioms of relating to and using analytic theories, especially contemporary Relational and Bionian theories, and, following from those differences, differences in how we each imagine the therapeutic relationship itself as an agent of change, especially as it evolves over time.
5 Wachtel (2014) also takes aim at the "left brain/right brain," and verbal/emotional dichotomies that I am calling into question. He cites both Damasio (1994) and LeDoux (2009) as taking the more holistic position that I am arguing for. Wachtel writes: "Rather than constituting separate realms, emotions and thoughts mutually create each other through reciprocal causal connections and neural pathways (Damasio, 1994). It is the essential unity of the two that is the foundation of human experience" (p. 424). Later he quotes LeDoux as saying: "the two sides [of the brain] are *closely interconnected and work together* in creating our mental and behavioral capacities . . . there is no overall function

of a side. . . . Systems span the brain vertically and horizontally—they are not isolated in one hemisphere" (p. 425).

6 The lesson that has remained with me from this groundbreaking paper was the courage Davies showed in revealing not only her momentary feelings of hatred toward the patient and herself but her *relationship to these feelings*—an openness to and acceptance of the truth of her emotional experience—thereby at least partially neutralizing her own shame, which, in turn, helped the patient feel less alone and ashamed, thereby dramatically opening and deepening the connection between them and the "conditions" in their analytic field more generally.

Chapter 6

The dialectic of empathy and freedom[1]

The concept of dialectical thinking or tension is a major subtext of contemporary Relational, constructivist and non-self-psychological intersubjective theory that, for the most part, has not been embraced by self psychology. Dialectical thinking has been central in the work of Mitchell (1993, 1997), Ogden (1986, 1994), Aron, 1996, Hoffman (1998), Benjamin (1988, 2004), and Bromberg (1998), to name only some of the more prominent authors to invoke the concept. I have argued that self psychology would benefit from incorporating a dialectical sensibility (S. Stern, 2004). While there are many dimensions of Relational dialectical theorizing,[2] the one I will be focusing on in this chapter is probably closest to Hoffman's (1998). Describing this dimension in my own words, I would say that the analyst's capacity to hold two opposing principles in mind simultaneously both opens and stabilizes the analytic space more than is possible when adhering to a single principle. In the present chapter I will attempt to make this argument in a more systematic and comprehensive way by applying dialectical logic to self psychology's most central therapeutic concept—analytic empathy. In so doing I hope to establish a more fundamental connection between self psychology and the other contemporary Relational theories with which it has been dynamically interacting.

Empathy: toward dialectical oppositions

Among the foundational concepts of self psychology, that of analytic empathy—the analyst's empathic inquiry, immersion, and attunement—has been the most central and enduring. Whereas Kohut's more metapsychological concepts, including the concept of the self, have gradually yielded to more experience-near, phenomenological, process-oriented constructions, all self psychologists continue to regard the analyst's efforts empathically to apprehend and comprehend the patient's subjective experience, and be guided in his interventions by that empathic understanding, as central to the self psychological approach to therapy.

We know from Kohut's (1959, 1982, 1984) repeated attempts to clarify what he meant by empathy that it is a complex concept. It has at least three meanings within the self psychology literature. It refers to the analyst's approach to data-gathering or listening. That is, the analyst seeks to listen to the patient's communications in an empathic (or, as Kohut put it, vicariously introspective) manner, actively attempting to understand the patient's experience from the patient's perspective. Empathy refers, secondly, to the analyst's interventions that attempt to convey the understanding gleaned from empathic listening. In this sense the analyst seeks to make empathic statements, or as Stolorow and Atwood (1992) have described them, statements that convey "validating attunement" to the patient's experience and affective states. And thirdly, empathy refers to the patient's experience of the analyst's efforts if they succeed. That is, the patient experiences the analyst's communications as empathic or attuned. In this last sense, empathy is not just something that is attempted: it is something that is actually achieved. It is the achievement of empathic communication that Kohut (1982) came to believe had curative potential. When we use the term empathy loosely, we often refer to all three of these processes at once, even though it is not necessarily the case that they always occur together. Empathy may be attempted, but not necessarily achieved. Conversely, empathy may be achieved without necessarily having been consciously sought or intended.

Some contemporary self-psychological theorists have come to feel that empathy, in any of these three meanings, is not a sufficient principle of analytic engagement and transformation (Bacal, 1998; Teicholz, 1999, 2000, 2006; Fosshage, 2003; Shane, 2006). Influenced by object relations theories, critiques of self psychology from Relational and constructivist authors (Mitchell, 1988, 1997; Hoffman, 1983, 1998; Bromberg, 1989; Slavin & Kriegman, 1992, 1998), and an evolving appreciation of the radically intersubjective nature of the analytic process that cuts across analytic schools, they have grappled with the questions raised and proposed a variety of creative responses, some of which move toward the dialectical sensibilities of the Relational theorists.

In the domain of analytic data gathering or listening, Fosshage (2003) has proposed what he terms the "other-centered listening position" to supplement the "empathic listening position." Within the other-centered position, the analyst shifts from empathic listening to a focus on the patient's affective impact on the analyst as a separate other, and does not necessarily seek to immediately convert this impact into empathic understanding. Rather, the analyst may elect tactfully to convey this affective impact to the patient as both a potentially useful form of feedback and an element of authentic exchange.

In the second empathic domain, expressed empathic understandings, a complex dialogue has been unfolding concerning the relationship between empathy and so-called analytic authenticity, or the analyst's expressive use of his own subjectivity (Teicholz, 1999, 2000; Orange, 2002; VanDerHeide, 2007)—the latter value being central to a Relational approach (Mitchell, 1988; Renik, 1993; Hoffman, 1998). While a full rendering of this discourse is beyond the scope of this chapter, my own sense is that there has been a paradoxical quality to the self-psychological arguments around the issue. On one hand, self psychologists have argued, in my view correctly, that empathy and authenticity constitute a false dichotomy because being empathic does not necessarily mean that one is being inauthentic (and vice versa) (Teicholz, 2000; Orange, 2002; VanDerHeide, 2007). On the other hand, it is recognized (at least implicitly) that were it not for the Relational critique, authenticity would probably not be coming up as a major concern for self psychologists. Although one can find references to authenticity in Kohut's writings (Teicholz, 1999, 2000), it was not a central thrust of his theory of technique. In this sense, self psychology is incorporating important aspects of Relational theory, and is clearly seeking to work out its own compromise with Relational technical values.

One form that compromise is taking follows the work of Slochower (1996) by locating the values of empathy and authenticity within a (primarily Winnicottian) developmental framework (Teicholz, 1999). Both Slochower and Teicholz recognize that empathy and authenticity don't always converge: there are times when the analyst's authentic subjectivity is "disjunctive" with the patient's current subjective experience or state, and the analyst faces a choice about whether or not to consciously, intentionally express his disjunctive experience. The answer from these authors is that it depends on the current state of the patient's self. Especially during early or regressed phases of treatment when the patient's self is presumed to be in a fragile, inchoate, or fragmented state, these authors feel the patient is not yet ready for a fully intersubjective interaction in which the analyst shares his subjective states, but rather needs the analyst to "hold" or "bracket" his own subjectivity and try to stay in a predominantly empathic mode. In this sense, disjunctive expressions of the analyst's subjectivity are viewed as appropriate to developmentally more mature, or at least more secure, forms of relating in which the patient can now tolerate and benefit from experiences of mutual as opposed to exclusively one-way recognition.

In a related vein, E. Shane (Shane, Shane & Gales, 1997; Shane, 2006) has suggested a developmental framework for listening and responding to the patient based on the analyst's assessment of the state of the patient's self. When the patient is primarily experiencing the analyst within the "self-transforming other dimension" the analyst seeks to be mindful of the various functions he is serving and intervene so as to foster the self-consolidation process. By contrast, when the patient is operating within the "interpersonal sharing other dimension," the analyst becomes freer to share his own subjectivity in the hope of fostering new experiences of "shared humanity, mutuality, affection, liking, and even love" (Shane, 2006, p. 28).

The technical oppositions of empathic vs. other-centered listening, empathic vs. authentic modes of participation, and self-transforming vs. interpersonal sharing dimensions of listening/responding could each be framed as dialectical oppositions in the sense meant by Relational theorists, and perhaps their authors intend them this way. But, as currently described, they are presented more as technical options carrying different therapeutic possibilities to be employed in different situations.[3] Hoffman (1998) adopted Ogden's (1986) definition of a dialectic as "*a process in which each of two opposing concepts creates, informs, preserves, and negates the other, each standing in a dynamic (ever changing) relationship with the other*" (p. 208, emphasis added). Hoffman has described such a dialectical relationship between analytic discipline and expressive spontaneity, and his argument *could* be applied to the opposition of empathy and authenticity. It could be argued, for example, that empathic listening and communication form a background and foundation against which the analyst's more spontaneous or authentic self-expressions derive particular therapeutic power; and conversely that the analyst's more self-contained empathic intentions become more powerful to the degree that the patient experiences the analyst as a real person who is responding to her in a unique, personal, authentic way. But self psychologists have not tended to formulate the principles of empathy and authenticity in this dialectical fashion.

The concept of freedom in Bion and Winnicott

These expanded technical models seek to address the limitations of certain aspects of the concept of empathy but, in my view, don't address the concept in its full depth or complexity. What is missed, or not fully stated, in these models is that sustained empathic inquiry/immersion/attunement is most fundamentally an *intention*, or to invoke Bion's (1967, 1970) language, a "desire". The self-psychological analyst *wants* to listen and speak empathically because he believes that empathic communication is what will be most therapeutic for the patient, and most facilitative of a deepening analytic process in which a progressive sense of safety and security will enable the patient to bring more of herself into the relationship and the dialogue. It is this premise that I believe needs closer scrutiny. In what follows I will argue that the intention to be analytically empathic needs to be held in dialectical tension with the (paradoxical) intention to participate in a way that is *free* of intention.

Bion (1962, 1970), a theorist in the Kleinian tradition whose ideas have found limited resonance with self psychologists, identified two kinds of necessary freedom—each associated with a different conceptual model and phase of his thinking (Ogden 2004). In his earlier model, organized around the concept of *container/contained*, the emphasis was on the analyst's capacity for *reverie*—a capacity to *process* all of the incoming information, not so much through conscious intention but through largely unconscious operations that have much in common with and are grounded in the analyst's primary process (Bion, 1962). The analyst must perform this function because, Bion believed, mothers of severely disturbed patients often have lacked this capacity, and therefore were unable to provide a sufficient *container* for the infant or young child's inchoate affects, impulses, and projections. Thus the child was left with certain *processing deficits* (in Bion's terminology, a deficit in *alpha function*). If one leaves out the Kleinian emphasis on projective identification in Bion's theory, the basic model of *container/contained* has much in common with the selfobject functions of self-psychological theory. Containment, defined as a mother's capacity to *hold and process* all that is stirred within her affectively and cognitively by her infant or young child, might well be understood as a selfobject function.

For Bion, the essence of the capacity for reverie was a kind of inner freedom. The mother or analyst needed to be able to receive and process all that was coming in as freely as possible, with no preconception of where the internal processing might lead, or what it might yield. In Bion's words:

> . . . reverie is that state of mind which is open to the reception of any "objects" from the loved object and is therefore capable of reception of the infant's projective identifications whether they are felt by the infant to be good or bad. In short, reverie is a factor of the mother's alpha-function.
>
> (1962, p. 36)

This is crucial analytically because part of what patients present are blockages or breakdowns of one kind or another in their own capacities to experience and process their most intense affective states (Eigen, 1996; Ogden, 2009). Often, corresponding blockages emerge in the analyst's own capacity to process and think, and it is the recognition of this blocked processing of affective experience, that is often the starting point for therapeutic movement.[4] Although ultimately the yield of the mother/analyst's reverie needs to be conveyed back to the child/patient empathically,[5] the internal processing itself is not constrained by the effort to be empathic.

Bion's (1967, 1970) later model was organized around his famous injunction to approach every analytic session "without memory or desire." Here, the emphasis is less on internal processing than on attention and apprehension, although clearly there are continuities in the sense that both have to do with the recognition and processing of emotional reality—especially its most disturbing forms. This model was reviewed in Chapter 3, so will not be recapitulated here. What I want to reemphasize in this context is that Bion was aiming for a kind of undirected attentional freedom—attention unencumbered by preconception (in which he included theoretical agendas and anything the analyst thinks he already knows about the patient), or any need the analyst might have in relation to the patient (including the need to cure her)—in order better to intuitively sense and perceive the true psychic reality of the patient and session at the moment.

Accordingly, from both of these Bionian perspectives, when a self psychological analyst enters the psychoanalytic space with a primary intention of listening and speaking empathically, and of providing experiences of validating attunement, he is entering with a preconceived, theoretically determined *desire* that will almost certainly interfere with the radical freedom necessary for apprehending and processing the current psychic reality of the session.

From a different theoretical sensibility, Winnicott placed freedom at the very center of his therapeutic values (Eigen, 1996). Like Kohut, Winnicott (1965) was preeminently concerned with maternal and analytic empathy. Especially with young infants, Winnicott believed mothers needed to be fully devoted to intuiting and responding to their children's needs, and in this sense had to sacrifice their own subjectivities in the service of their children *for a while.* But starting when the child was still fairly young, Winnicott (1969) believed the dynamic had to shift gradually such that the mother made sure to "survive" as a person under the pressures of the child's needs, projections and omnipotent demands. Empathy has to become balanced by a certain kind of self-integrity. Not only is this essential for the mother, it is also crucial for the child's self-development. If the mother can't survive as an individual, she also won't be strong enough to carry the child through the child's own developmental processes to becoming a self capable of recognizing, relating to, and surviving among other selves. In Winnicott's vision of both childhood and analysis there is always the understanding that the dyad in question has to *go through something together*; if both parties come out intact, development can proceed.

Surviving for Winnicott was tantamount to the safeguarding of inner freedom—specifically the freedom to be oneself in the presence of the other. Conversely, the loss of this freedom was tantamount to psychic death. A patient with a false self was a patient who had sacrificed this crucial inner freedom out of the need to comply with parental requirements—a formulation very close to Brandchaft's (1994, Brandchaft et al., 2010) later theory of pathological accommodation. In analysis, Winnicott (1965) tried to provide a holding environment that offered the patient the necessary intersubjective space within which to begin to reclaim the freedom to be oneself in the presence of the other. This is not unlike Brandchaft's effort to offer a milieu in which the patient can "free the spirit from its cell." But, unlike Brandchaft, Winnicott (1969) believed that empathic understanding alone was not a sufficient therapeutic principle to create such a therapeutic space. Some patients—those who have not yet achieved "object usage"— begin analysis relating to the analyst "through identifications": i.e., through transferences, projections, early identifications, and unconscious control operations that constitute a kind of assault on the analyst's selfhood and analytic functioning. Only by recognizing this negation, and taking steps to combat or free himself from it, can the analyst become a "useable object." Thus the analyst's capacity ultimately to exercise his *freedom to function analytically, whatever that might mean in a given case*, is crucial for the establishment of a potential space in which the patient can reclaim her own freedom to be. To quote Winnicott (1962): "In doing psycho-analysis I aim at: Keeping alive; Keeping well; Keeping awake. I aim at being myself . . . " (p. 166).

This formulation of Winnicott's, as carried forward by theorists such as Bollas (1987), Ogden (1994, 1997), and Benjamin (1988), has been enormously influential in contemporary Relational psychoanalysis. In its contemporary versions the model loses the unidirectional quality of Kleinian theory (which Winnicott was starting to move away from anyway) and recognizes that the patient does not literally invade or put something into the analyst's mind. Rather, it is understood that the analyst unconsciously participates in the creation of his own countertransference (Ogden, 1994). As I have previously suggested (S. Stern, 2004), countertransference is best approached dialectically—that is, the analyst assumes a complex interplay between his own and the patient's contributions to the countertransference. Understandings and interpretations are reached from a position that tries to keep this tension in mind.

I return to Bion and Winnicott in part because their theories underpin contemporary Relational and intersubjective theory, but primarily because their original thinking illuminates a central point I wish to make about analytic freedom. While there are a number of notable exceptions to the following generalization (see especially Symington, 1983; Eigen, 1996; Ogden, 1994, 1997), contemporary Relational theorists tend to stress the *expressive* dimension of analytic freedom. When Bollas (1987) writes about "expressive use of the countertransference," when Hoffman (1998) writes about "throwing away the book" and "spontaneity," when Mitchell (1988) and Ehrenberg (1992) write about "authenticity," when Ringstrom (2001, 2007) writes about "improvisation," or, in general, when Relationalists write about the analyst's expressive use of subjectivity, they focus primarily on things the analyst *says and does (in a technical sense)* and frame this expressive participation as being in dialectical tension with analytic discipline and restraint—i.e., the conventional inhibitions on what the analyst says and does. Self psychologists, influenced by these theorists, pick up on this emphasis and speak of authenticity as a technical choice that (under certain circumstances) stands in contrast with empathic interventions. I think that something of the profundity of Bion's and Winnicott's original formulations gets lost in this emphasis on technique. Both Bion and Winnicott were, I believe, at least as concerned with *the inner qualities of the analyst's mind-at-work* as they were with the analyst's technical choices and innovations. More than self-expression per se, they were concerned with the analyst's capacity to inhabit the psychic spaces that opened up (or closed down) in interactions with the patient, and then to be able to do what was necessary to remain "alive" analytically.

Moreover, analytic freedom is a more robust principle than the relational freedom to express one's subjectivity, because freedom in the Bionian or Winnicottian senses includes the freedom *not to* express one's subjectivity. (VanDerHeide, 2007, has made a similar point about analytic authenticity.) Thus, Winnicott (1969), later in his career, exercised his freedom from classical technical imperatives by deliberately not saying much with many of his patients, seeking to create a space in which they could more freely come to their own "interpretations." Similarly, Bion (1970) argued that one of the reasons for trying to suspend "memory and desire" was to be able to apprehend that which was *not yet known* about the patient's essential struggles. In this sense, freedom inhered in an unspoken quality of inquiry and receptivity.

The importance of this freedom not to act, or what I think of as *freedom of stillness* (as opposed to *freedom of movement* or self-expression), is highlighted by the contemporary understanding of relational trauma. One of the legacies of severe relational trauma is the enormous difficulty of simply experiencing one's feelings (S. Stern, 2002b, 2015; Stolorow, 2006). Bion's theory of container/contained addressed this problem, but we now have a richer intersubjective contextualization of it. The traumatized patient feels too alone, yet, paradoxically, too much at the mercy of the Other from whom she does not feel entirely differentiated, simply to "be with" her own feelings, recognized (mentalized) as such (Shaw, 2014; S.Stern, In preparation). So often, a feature of relational trauma is the systematic invalidation, repudiation, and/or projective distortion of the child's affective experience, making it psychologically impossible for the child (and later the adult patient) to experience her feelings in a way that anchors her to, and enables her to "use," her own subjective reality (S. Stern, 2002a, b, 2015, In preparation). The patient is unable to tolerate the very feelings she needs to feel in order to process her trauma, grieve it, and achieve a level of intersubjectivity (in Benjamin's developmental sense; see endnote 1) necessary for a greater sense of aliveness. Instead, the patient engages in various forms of externalization, identificatory confusion (Ferenczi, 1933; S. Stern, 2002a, b, 2015), dissociation, tendencies toward action, and desperate control operations that often have the effect of constraining or deadening the analytic space, and/or provoking repetitive enactments even as she may be trying to evoke new, needed responses from the analyst (S. Stern, 1994, 2002b). In response to all of this the analyst needs some greater capacity to "stay with" whatever is happening, especially whatever affects are lurking in the background or subtly destabilizing the patient and the relationship in the moment, and simply allow all of it to affect him, guide his reverie, and ultimately inform his interventions.

Historically, analysts have long-appreciated the freedom not to act—the effort to "sit still" and process—but were hampered in this by a one-person psychology that failed to alert them to their own inevitable participation in the two-way mutual-influence system of the analytic relationship. Now, paradoxically, our awareness of the *limits* of our freedom not to act potentially enhances that freedom by allowing us to consider our own participation in the creation of the present intersubjective moment. We now understand that part of what we may need to stay with is our own intolerable affects, emerging from our own histories of relational trauma and reactivated in the current analytic situation.

Our freedom not to act has also been impeded by the historical restrictions on the freedom *to* act. Paradoxically, only now that we feel freer *to act* (e.g., to be more personally expressive) when it seems necessary are we freer *not to act* and have that inaction be a true expression of freedom rather than a defensive clinging to a stereotype of the analytic role. It is not coincidental that Winnicott (1949) was one of first analysts to give himself the freedom to speak the countertransference, *and* (1969) one of the first to give himself the freedom not to speak at all for long periods of time.

The dialectic of empathy and freedom

Taking Bion's and Winnicott's theories as points of departure, I have come to regard analytic freedom as a core ideal for the analyst's working subjectivity, and a necessary dialectical counterpart to analytic empathy. Like analytic empathy, analytic freedom could be described as a quality of the analyst's listening, sensing, and processing; of the analyst's speaking and acting; or of the effect on the patient (and the analyst) of the analyst's exercise of freedom. (See also Chapter 3.) However, as with empathy, I suggest that in the fullest sense of the term it refers to an intention or core value or ideal. Analytic freedom as a core value is not encumbered by the intention to be analytically empathic. In this sense, to use a Winnicottian word, the analyst's exercise of freedom must be *ruthless*. However, I view analytic empathy as an equally important core value, and as existing in constant dialectical tension with analytic freedom. It may seem to be semantic quibbling, contradictory, or confusing to say that the analyst needs to be unencumbered by the "desire" to be empathic while at the same time holding empathy in mind constantly as part of a dialectical process. I would argue that it is a necessary paradox. We do aim to be empathic, *ultimately*. Patients do need to feel understood and that we are deeply committed to understanding them. But such understanding cannot be forced or rushed (Bollas, 1987; Bromberg, 1989; Ehrenberg, 1992; Ogden, 1994, 1997), and the analyst needs to feel free to experience *whatever* he is experiencing and use that experience to further the analytic process in whatever way seems most promising.

The larger point, however, is that there is more going on in a productive analytic process than the communication and achievement of empathy. The patient and analyst, in a unique and circumscribed way, *create a life together*—a life whose purpose is to help the patient work out a better life, or, as it often subjectively feels to the patient, have a life at all (Ehrenberg, 1992; Eigen, 1996; Ogden, 1997; Stolorow, 2006). That co-created life is multi-dimensional, and it is this lived, co-created life in its totality that the patient draws upon in reanimating and recreating her own life. The patient looks to the analyst to navigate and take primary responsibility for moving (or at least pointing) their relationship, and ultimately the patient, toward life. Of course, paradoxes abound here, because the analyst is always following (empathically), even as he is leading. But in order to perform his function as leader he needs to be able to stay alive, which requires the exercise of analytic freedom: always inwardly, sometimes inwardly and outwardly at the same time.

I would even argue that the capacity for analytic empathy *rests* on the various capacities involved in analytic freedom. If one does not experience some "freedom of movement," or have the capacity to recognize, and ultimately take steps to emerge from, restrictions on this freedom, the capacity for empathy will be impaired by the sense of imprisonment within co-created transference-countertransference frames or worlds. And if one does not have some "freedom of stillness"—the freedom to "sit still" and simply "be with" whatever is happening affectively, both internally and in the room—one is constantly at risk of getting caught up in the patient's defensive or enactive solutions to problems of affect tolerance and regulation, thereby losing the capacity to empathize with the patient's underlying affect states and desperate need to avoid experiencing them. As Stolorow (personal communication) concisely stated it: "The analyst's experiential freedom is a condition for the possibility of empathic-introspective inquiry."

This is not to say that the analyst can ever escape the constant shaping influence of intersubjective context, including the contribution of his own personal history (Atwood & Stolorow, 1984). Analytic freedom is always limited and relative. Like empathy, it is never complete and never "immaculate" (Stolorow, 1993; personal communication). The most dramatic evidence of this is the inevitability of enactments. Enactments involve, almost by definition, a curtailment of both the analyst's freedom *and* empathic capacities. But, by dint of training, theory, personal analysis, experience, and the potential resources available to him in relation to his work, the analyst, we hope, possesses a *processing capacity*—one might think of it as a special form of hard-won wisdom—that gives him *relative* freedom, or at least potential freedom, to think and move (or "sit still and stay with") even within these highly pressurized analytic spaces. Indeed, the trend in contemporary theory toward the analyst's radical self-reflectivity—the attempt to be open to, reflect on, and make use of, one's total subjectivity when in the presence of the patient—deepens our capacity for analytic freedom in just such pressurized intersubjective spaces.[6]

In concluding this section I would say that occupying the dialectic of empathy and freedom is stabilizing for the analyst, and ultimately for both parties—like trying to keep one's balance using two feet rather than one, or locating oneself geographically using two coordinates rather than one. Empathy alone leaves too much intersubjective territory out of view. Freedom alone opens intersubjective spaces but is too unbounded to be a sufficient therapeutic principle. Together they expand and contain each other. The tension between them is highly generative: It brings the analytic process fully to life.

The cutting edge of intersubjective clinical data: Linda and me[7]

I began seeing Linda, a happily married woman in her early fifties who had been in long-term, once-a-week, therapy with various therapists throughout much of her adult life. She was, in fact, devoted to self-improvement and went to many weekend and week-long therapeutic workshops in addition to her primary therapy. During the first year of her twice-weekly therapy with me she seemed quite engaged during many of her sessions. She was articulately self-reflective, was firmly present and focused in the here-and-now, back-and-forth of our exchange, and, despite her own self-experience to the contrary, had a self-assured presence that I sensed others in her life also felt. Yet, paradoxically, there was often a palpable feeling of anxiety in the room. There was also a sense that whatever deepening engagement or understanding or relaxation might be achieved in a given session, by the next session it felt like we were starting all over again, just as anxiously. She also missed many sessions as a matter of course, mostly due to other therapeutic experiences she scheduled for herself, but also frequent vacations. These breaks in the continuity of our sessions added to the feeling of starting over each time.

An aspect of my own subjectivity in this treatment was that Linda was one of my first patients following my relocation to Portland, Maine, after practicing twenty years in Chicago. Consequently, I felt much more reticent about establishing my usual psychoanalytic frame. I was now working in a regional culture that was relatively unfamiliar with, and suspicious of, psychoanalysis, and I was still getting my bearings. It seemed that the therapeutic culture in Maine had a more new age quality: Many people sought the kinds of brief, intensive, therapeutic experiences that Linda was pursuing. I had passing thoughts that maybe psychoanalysis really is old fashioned, and I need to get up to speed in the same way that I need to get up to speed on the computer! Plus, I liked Linda and didn't want to scare her away. So, I was uncharacteristically passive and permissive regarding these absences, contenting myself to try to explore their meaning through attempted empathic inquiry.

I learned a lot in this way. I came to understand Linda's extreme anxiety about dependence—her suspiciousness of, and fear of being exploited or controlled by, authority figures. She could acknowledge that this was operating between us. She didn't trust me in a general way, even if there were sessions when she liked things I said. I also learned about her lifelong drive for self-improvement. She lived with deep feelings of defectiveness and felt she had to be constantly doing things to improve or progress or she would fall into a kind of ontological sloth, accompanied by self-hatred. Thus, the many workshops and retreats had an almost compulsive quality. Yet they were always, legitimately, very powerful experiences for her. Somehow, in the group setting, away from her familiar intersubjective world, in the aura of a charismatic facilitator, she was able to come more alive and experience seemingly transformative interactions with others or with herself in the group context. She would invariably return from them with an inner glow—a glow, I was aware, she almost never experienced in her sessions with me. In fact, because of my relatively non-directive approach, I believe Linda experienced many of her sessions with me as a kind of echo chamber for her feelings of stuckness and deadness. Thus, her therapy came to feel to her like a prison, and a break for any reason was a relief. This sense was further reinforced by the fact that, in addition to her frequent absences, she also fell into a pattern of coming five to ten minutes late to her sessions. When we talked about any of this she was always interested; it got her attention. And she would try to reform for a while. But improvements were short-lived.

What I want to emphasize here is that my psychoanalytic subjectivity with Linda began to be split between two levels. At one level I was operating in the mode of empathic-introspective inquiry, trying to stay with her subjective experience and trying to understand it. I *was* coming to understand her better, and at times she was clearly impressed and moved by my understanding. A haunting picture of her mother as an anxiously, deadeningly controlling figure, had begun to emerge. Linda had survived psychologically by distancing herself from her mother. Thus, I began to understand intellectually why I felt cast into an odd kind of non-existence, as if Linda were saying, "It's nothing personal, but when I'm not here you don't exist, and truthfully I'd rather not be here . . . but then, part of me must want to be here sometimes or I wouldn't come." Despite my growing understanding, at another level I could feel hurt, insecure, frustrated, angry, and helpless (in part, undoubtedly, reflecting my own history of insecure attachments)—all mixed with my liking of Linda and a sense of connection, or potential connection, with her. There seemed to be no bridging the two levels—at least not for very long. Empathy and insight were not leading to behavior change, and my deepening understanding was not helping me with my feelings when she would miss sessions. I began to worry that perhaps Linda's instincts were right: Perhaps the workshops worked well for her, whereas the therapy was pulling her toward a malignant regression against which she was wisely defending herself.

I think of my situation with Linda as a dramatic example of what I might call *the cutting edge of intersubjective clinical data.* I'm trying to capture with this phrase a number of interrelated qualities or dimensions of the lived psychoanalytic interaction from the analyst's perspective. First is the nonlinear, unpredictable, ever-changing nature of the intersubjective interaction, which requires a kind of openness and freedom on the part of the analyst as he attempts to keep up with and register all that is going on at "the cutting edge" of the interaction and of his moment-to-moment experience/understanding of the patient. A second quality is the fact that the data under scrutiny are always, inescapably, intersubjective (Stolorow et al., 1987). That is, the analyst is always a participant in the very data under observation, and in that sense the data are always in part *lived* experience. At this level, the analyst strives to be free in the sense of abandoning or surrendering himself to that lived experience rather than trying to control or stand outside it. He also, simultaneously, seeks to observe and process that lived experience, as he also considers the patient's evolving subjectivity in the context of their co-created lived experience. A third quality is that, because we enter this intimate intersubjective space with people who live with traumatic inner struggles, and invite them to bring those struggles "into the room," the nature of the intersubjective data we encounter is often deeply disturbing, disorienting, threatening, enveloping and imprisoning. It has a "cutting edge" and that edge is often not something we can comfortably sit back, observe, and empathize with. It is vivid, real, lived experience, and it often demands some kind of response, lest the analysis stagnate, or worse. At this level, it can have the quality of a protracted "now moment" (D.N. Stern et al., 1998), and the question is what to do with it. At this level the interaction calls for freedom in the sense of responding creatively and uniquely to the particular struggle being enacted, especially when the struggle has the effect of restricting or impairing freedom in some way. In systems theory terms, one might say freedom is needed to perturb traumatically informed attractor states. Empathic statements can work in many situations, but they need to carry the force of a lived, authentic response that emerges from what is really happening intersubjectively (Geist, 2007). Perhaps someone more skilled in the art of empathic imagining could have reached Linda through empathic statements. I could not.

As Linda and I were approaching our first summer of work together, she brought out her calendar at the beginning of a session and said she wanted to talk about our summer schedule. She let me know that between various workshops and vacations she would be missing the equivalent of about five weeks of sessions during the summer. I knew at that point that I had to say something, and the question was, what to say. It took me a few minutes to gather myself. I tried to process as best I could all that had been gathering in me over the past year. I chose my words carefully, but they were completely heartfelt. I said:

> I have to tell you—I don't like it when you miss so many sessions. I could say that I don't think it's good for your therapy to miss so much, and that would be the truth. I do think that. I could say more about my understanding of why you miss so much, and what I think you're scared of, but we've already talked about that. I could say that we need to establish more of a clear structure around cancellations, which we do. But I realize that the more basic thing is, I don't *like* it when you miss sessions. I wish you would come more consistently.

Linda sat up and looked at me in a way she never had before. She was clearly stunned by what I had said and the way I had said it. She asked me to say more about why I didn't like it. I told her I couldn't say too much more than I already had. I admitted I especially didn't like it when she went to other therapy experiences. She said, "You don't?" I said, "No, I don't." She asked me to say more about why I didn't think it was good for her therapy to miss so much. I told her I didn't think she would find out what was possible in our therapy unless she made more of a commitment to show up for it. I said that I knew the workshops and retreats she attended felt enlivening in a way that therapy didn't, but that the difficult feelings in therapy would always be waiting for her and needed to be faced. I said I now knew her well enough to say that the effects of the workshops were always short-lived, and that she always drifted back to the feelings of depression and deadness that haunted her and were the reason she was in therapy. I said I thought that only by coming to therapy, no matter what, would she be able to find out if therapy could really help her with that.

Her immediate association was to feeling seduced, but added that that wasn't necessarily a bad thing. She then associated to her sexuality—something we had scarcely talked about—and said she was aware that her sexuality had been deadened for a long time and that, even though it was a frightening subject to contemplate talking about with me, she wanted to try to do that. Over the next few weeks Linda talked about her commitment to therapy. She acknowledged that she had been hedging her bets, and vowed to participate more whole-heartedly for at least a year to see if what I was saying was true. It wasn't that she trusted me, she made sure to clarify, but felt she owed it to me and the therapy to at least try to do it in the way I thought would have the best chance of working. During this same period, I proposed, and she agreed to, a new policy about missed sessions.

In the two years since this confrontation Linda has faithfully kept to her commitment, and the therapy has deepened considerably. In retrospect, she admits that during the first year she experienced her new commitment as in part an obligation she was performing because she had experienced me as insisting on it—i.e., a partial enactment of a maternal transference. In her words, "I felt like I had been sent to jail." However, she has increasingly experienced the commitment as a choice *she* is making, and one that has paid off significantly. Initially, living with the feelings of inner deadness, without going off for an infusion of borrowed life, was extremely depressing for Linda. At times the sessions felt like torture to her—a torture she wanted to retreat from by going to sleep, or going home. Often, her defensive fatigue in sessions was palpable, and I would begin to yawn and get tired along with her. I learned to use my fatigue as a signal that she was approaching some extremely anxiety-provoking repressed or dissociated feelings and was defensively turning away from them. Gradually, she has developed greater tolerance for her frightening feelings, especially sadness and rage: She can now experience them glancingly, though not yet in a sustained way. These micro-shifts in sessions have been accompanied by more obvious improvements in her self-awareness and self-confidence outside of sessions.

Even as these improvements have evolved, however, there has been a continuation of Linda's pattern of emotional presence followed by withdrawal. In response to this unpredictability, I have entered many sessions with the anxiety that, once again, I would be encountering someone whom I barely knew and who might even decide to take a break for a while. There were some sessions—even strings of sessions—in which it felt like our relationship—our *attachment*—was, in fact, becoming more real and dependable, and I would begin to believe this was so. But then, unpredictably, she would come in and it was as if we were near-strangers again, and *this* was the truer reality of our situation. I would then react with self-doubt and insecurity, once again anxious that the thread holding us together could break or unravel at any moment. I *would* recognize that this was happening, and at times would comment on it. And talking about it usually led to a greater sense of shared understanding and conviction regarding Linda's anxiety about dependence, and her need to keep a foot out the door. But these moments of recognition were not proof against future repetitions of the whole sequence.

An aspect of my reverie around this repetitive pattern was a dawning awareness that the parental dimension of countertransference that I feel in one form or another with many of my longer-term patients was missing with Linda. Or more precisely, no sooner would I start to feel it than her withdrawal would make me feel like I had been presumptuous. This sense would be reinforced if I made any reference to child-to-parent aspects of Linda's transference, for example, interpreting her conflict around allowing herself to feel attached to me. Even if she acknowledged the existence of such a conflict, her discomfort would be apparent. These movements gradually, paradoxically, led to a *silent* freeing up of something in me such that I began to be able to *predict* Linda's recurring pattern of connection and withdrawal, began taking it less personally, and began feeling more open to Linda's shifting transference states. It was as if, simultaneously, I had accepted the possibility that Linda could push me away at any moment, *and* begun to feel more confident that, despite her withdrawals, she and I were becoming more attached.[8] Rather than approaching our sessions with the usual anxiety, I started feeling more secure and welcoming, as if I were now silently performing a kind of holding or containing function, and was actually curious in a positive sense about what I would encounter next. The causes of this shift in me seem somewhat mysterious. I attribute them mainly to my reverie process, both conscious and unconscious, but assume that process was cocreated in ways that also remain mysterious.

This movement in the transference-countertransference reached a spontaneous climax when Linda and I resumed recently after a long summer break. Soon into the first session she was talking about feeling quite distant, describing how she had thought very little about me during the break, as if I hardly existed for her. She felt more acutely disturbed and worried by this than usual, and asked me if I was feeling something similar. Immediately, with a smile, I said, "No, just the opposite: I'm feeling like I know you all too well!" She smiled broadly, relaxed her body, and expressed profound reassurance and pleasure that I had said this and obviously meant it. It took a few minutes for her to realize and say that at the moment I said this she felt reconnected with me. We were, it seemed, co-weaving the gold of more secure attachment from the straw of our co-created insecure attachment. Or were we!

As this session dramatizes, Linda has been developing an appetite for talking about our relationship, and things tend to feel livelier when she does. Compared to where we started, the transference is now not only in the room but in our dialogue. There are sessions when she asks me direct questions about my life, or psychoanalysis, and I have come to feel it is important to answer her most of the time. I view this as one way *she* is acting bolder and freer—actively seeking information that will help her assess my trustworthiness. Some months before the above-mentioned long summer break, she was asking about psychoanalysis and about how often I saw my other patients. I told her, and she asked if I ever thought of seeing her more often. In fact, I had been thinking about this over the previous few weeks and told her so. I said I had been thinking it might be good for her to increase because it would likely help her confront her fears of dependency. She was surprisingly intrigued, felt it was significant that we had somehow both come to this question at the same time, and promised to consider the possibility seriously over the next few months. It was actually in the post-vacation session described above, following my remark about knowing her all too well, that she announced her decision to increase to three sessions per week. Also recently, two years after my confrontation of her absences, it came to light that as a girl of about 12 she lost her father's attention to her younger brothers, had turned away from him emotionally to protect herself, and had felt profoundly hurt that he never seemed to notice her withdrawal, and never reached out to her or showed the same interest in her again.

I present this selective synopsis of Linda's and my analytic relationship because I believe it demonstrates the dialectical interplay of analytic empathy and analytic freedom, and the therapeutic yield of this dialectic over time. One might imagine or argue that a more consistently empathic stance could have worked just as well or better with Linda. For example, had I been more assertive about establishing my usual analytic frame with respect to missed sessions, and then tried empathically to respond to Linda's experience of those limits, perhaps things would have opened up in the treatment more quickly or less traumatically.

My own conviction about it is that saying what I did to Linda was extremely important, and that its therapeutic effect was in part immediate but in part progressive over time. While it is true that what I said was an authentic expression of my subjectivity, I don't think of that as exactly the therapeutic agent. For one thing, I don't think of what I said as being exactly "disjunctive," or unempathic with Linda's subjectivity, as Fosshage (2003) or Teicholz (1999) might construe it. I think of our subjectivities as having become intertwined in a particular way, and that when I said what I did it registered with Linda as both emerging from and addressing something she had played a part in. Nor do I think of what transpired between Linda and me as exactly an enactment; or at least its status as an enactment doesn't go to the heart of the experience for me. Enactment implies something unconscious or dissociated on the part of both parties (McLaughlin, 1991; Bromberg, 1998, 2006; D.B. Stern, 2010). I think I was more or less aware of what was happening but for a long time felt perplexed about what to do about it.

I do think of my confrontation of Linda's absences as an "act of freedom" (Symington, 1983), but I don't think the exercise of freedom came only at the point when I spoke up. It had been there all along in my willingness to experience and reflect upon my reactive affects without having to immediately express them. There is a paradox here, because I did, in another sense, feel un-free—un-free to establish my usual and preferred structure for dealing with missed sessions, and un-free to express my feelings as they were happening. Yet, I think I hesitated for reasons—my intuitive/empathic sense of what she and I were ready to handle together. Thus, there was, paradoxically, both a paralysis and a freedom (or perhaps, in the terms set forth in this paper, a dialectical tension between empathy and freedom) expressed in my choice *not* to say anything until the moment I did. (Can one feel free to feel un-free?) Moreover, I have continued to exercise freedom in various less dramatic ways since our confrontation: for example, being open to my fatigue and using it to ground my responses to Linda's resistance to experiencing her painful affects; the relatively silent freeing up that has occurred surrounding the central transference-countertransference negotiation of our attachment relationship; my spontaneous joke about that; and finally, feeling free to answer Linda's direct questions about me.

Self-transformation reconsidered

Self psychological analysts are concerned with changing the patient's experience of self and self-with-other. How does this come about? The answers to this question have grown more varied and complex along with our theories. Kohut's self psychology was both a deficit and a developmental arrest theory; hence self-transformation was thought of as a developmental process set in motion by the patient's progressive experience of the analyst as a needed selfobject. Still operating within a classically influenced metapsychology and theory of technique, Kohut (1984) insisted that his was not a theory advocating direct gratification of needs but rather of structural growth through optimal frustration, transmuting internalization, and empathic self-understanding that was the product of self-psychologically informed interpretations. Yet, he straddled the fence, and at times (e.g., 1984) crossed over and acknowledged that successful analyses were also corrective new emotional experiences. Perhaps we would say that by the end Kohut had evolved to a dialectical position with respect to therapeutic action—struggling to hold a psychoanalytic frame oriented toward empathic understanding and interpretation while at the same time beginning to recognize that a needed emotional connection between analyst and analysand, however that might be achieved, was also essential. In hindsight, it seems to me that this generative dialectical tension in Kohut's legacy has fostered and shaped the subsequent theoretical developments in contemporary self psychology.

The rudiments of this dialectical tension go at least as far back in psychoanalysis as Strachey (1934), who understood that mutative transference interpretations were effective both for their content and because they offered a new transformative interpersonal experience (see Gill, 1982).

For Strachey, this was the experience of a less harsh superego that the analysand could internalize. The idea that the analyst could accomplish both things at once—understanding and new experience—has been very persistent. We still see this ideal operating in both Gill's (1982) and Kohut's (1984) revolutionary reformulations of the analytic process. But the literature on analytic freedom has gradually clarified that the two principles or processes at times operate separately and dialectically rather than always simultaneously or isomorphically. It has pulled the principles of empathic understanding and new lived experience apart and said, in effect, that the analyst must be free to draw upon his total subjectivity, not just his empathic intentions, as he listens, feels, processes, speaks, and acts within the intersubjective analytic space.

This understanding in turn rests on the more fundamental dialectic between individual subjectivity and dyadic intersubjectivity wherein the two dimensions of experience are continually constituting each other in infinitely complex ways (Mitchell, 1988; Ogden, 1994; Stolorow, 1997b).[9] It is not only the analyst's empathic grasp of the patient's subjectivity that leads to self-transformation. It is the total lived intersubjective relationship that is transformative. Thus, although I did not fully understand the significance of my intervention at the time, I believe it was Linda's experience of my wanting and pursuing her in the face of her self-protective withdrawal, unlike her father, and expressing my wishes and intentions directly (rather than indirectly trying to control her), unlike her mother, that began to transform her sense of the kind of engagement that was possible between us, and opened her horizon to the possibility of facing rather than escaping her most painful feelings. Once it is fully understood that self-transformation occurs within, and in response to, the total intersubjective relationship, the door is opened for self psychologists to embrace analytic freedom as the necessary dialectical partner of analytic empathy in the analysis of the self.

Notes

1 This chapter is a shortened and slightly revised version of my paper by the same name published in *The International Journal of Psychoanalytic Self Psychology* (2009, *Volume 4*: 132–164). The revisions are mainly in my summary of Bion's ideas, reflecting my greater immersion in his work since writing the original paper. The conceptual sections of the present chapter expand on themes first introduced in the final section of Chapter 3.

2 It is beyond the scope of this chapter to fully develop the following, but I would propose a distinction between at least three kinds of dialectic that have emerged in the Relational literature: *existential*, *developmental,* and *technical*. An *existential* dialectic is one that is inherent in the human condition (or in a particular domain of human experience), and over which one has little or no control. Ogden (1994) regards the relationship between the Freudian conscious and unconscious as the first such dialectic to have been discovered and named within psychoanalysis. That is, according to Ogden, the revolutionary insight in Freud's topographical model is that human subjectivity is constituted dialectically in the complex interplay of conscious and unconscious experience. Teicholz (1999) has argued that the relationship between self and selfobject in Kohut's theory is another such dialectic: the experiences of self and selfobject connectedness are understood to be mutually constitutive aspects of human subjectivity. An example of a *developmental* dialectic is Benjamin's (1988, 1990) dialectic between self-assertion and recognition of the other's subjectivity. The capacity to shift back and forth between one and the other, and to fully appreciate their essential interdependence, is a developmental achievement rather than a human given. Finally, the various dialectical tensions identified by Hoffman (1998) as guides for the analyst's therapeutic presence or intentionality are examples of *technical* dialectics. The dialectics between, for example, expressive spontaneity and analytic discipline, or relational mutuality and asymmetry, refer to more or less conscious aspects of the analyst's intentionality or technique that, if recognized and embraced, are thought to contribute to therapeutic action. There may be, in addition, hybrid or more complex forms of dialectic. For example, the relationship between self and interactive regulation in Beebe and Lachmann's (2002) work strikes me as a complex dialectic with elements of all three types (although they, themselves, do not label it a dialectic). While I believe all three forms have potential contributions to make within self psychology, it is the last type that I will be focusing on in this chapter.

3 Teicholz (personal communication) has alerted me to an important, though unpublished, paper of hers in which she does fully embrace a dialectical relationship between empathy and authenticity (Teicholz, 2002). Thus, my statement here refers only to her published positions on the topic.

4 We see these ideas carried forward in the work of Eigen (1996) and Ogden (1994) as well as in the contemporary Relational understanding of enactment as a mutual or shared dissociation (Bromberg, 1998; D.B. Stern, 2003).

5 See Waddell (1998) for a beautiful rendering of Bion's developmental theory, replete with vivid examples of both mother-infant and therapist-patient interactions illustrating reverie and containment functions.

6 Though beyond the scope of the present paper, it occurs to me that the analyst's exercise of relative freedom is a primary basis for the patient's development of an idealizing selfobject transference. Idealization is a complex topic: I believe there are many forms of it. Some forms are "given;" some are "earned." It is the earned idealization that, I believe, is ultimately most therapeutic. One of the

principal ways the analyst earns the patient's necessary idealization is through the competent exercise of analytic freedom.

7 The subject of this clinical narrative is the same patient (and treatment) presented as the illustrative example at the end of Chapter 1. The present account was written and published at about year 4 of Linda's 9-year analysis. It is strongly suggested that the reader re-consider the condensed overview in Chapter 1 after reading this more detailed, in-depth rendering of the process.

8 Benjamin (2004), following Ghent (1990), has described this as surrender, on the analyst's part, to the "intersubjective third." It also seems to have qualities of the shift toward mentalization described by Fonagy et al. (2002).

9 The dialectic of subjectivity and intersubjectivity falls in the category of *existential* dialectics, which I defined in note 1.

Chapter 7

The conundrum of self-care

Introduction: two kinds of need

Before beginning the essay that constitutes the main body of this chapter, I want to set it in a larger meta-theoretical framework that connects it to the themes of this book. The concept of needed relationship contains an inherent ambiguity: On one hand it implies a provision of some kind that addresses a *felt need* of the patient's; on the other hand, it is ultimately the analyst's responsibility to determine what kind of relational engagement is needed to facilitate the patient's movement toward his implicit, evolving therapeutic-developmental aims.[1] In this sense, the needed relationship is both "of the patient" and "of the analyst." Sometimes, these two reverberating dimensions of needed relationships are in relative harmony or congruence: That which the patient feels he needs (even if unconsciously) has significant correspondence with that which the analyst also senses he needs. In other situations, however, things can become much more complex and murky. With my patient Linda (presented in Chapters 1 and 6), for example, my strong conviction that she *needed* a more consistent and intensive analytic immersion was at odds with her *felt need* to control and limit our connection, always keeping one foot out the door. Yet, this apparent conflict was murky because of the aims she had clearly set for herself (and us) in the first session of the analysis, which, in the end, she was thrilled to have been able to achieve to the degree that she did.

Although not framing this duality in the same way I have, Gedo (1979) is the main psychoanalytic theorist to have approached the topic (or one close to it) in a systematic way. Writing in the late 1970s, Gedo was seeking to develop a comprehensive therapeutic approach that addressed not only the problems of the Oedipal neuroses, but of pre-Oedipal developmental arrests that had been elaborated theoretically in the work Winnicott,

Balint, Loewald, Kohut, George Klein and others. Building on earlier work done in collaboration with Goldberg (Gedo & Goldberg, 1973), he identified five "modes" of treatment, each corresponding to different levels in a developmental hierarchy of psychological functioning. Of these five therapeutic modes, only modes 4 and 5 (the most advanced) addressed problems that were "located" within the patient's subjective, phenomenological experience; whereas modes 1, 2, and 3 all pertained to what Gedo called "objective needs"—earlier needs that he regarded as "organismic" and therefore not amenable to introspection or to a predominantly interpretive technical approach. Unlike felt needs and wishes and their associated intrapsychic conflicts, which, as an aspect of unconscious subjectivity, could be expressed through the patient's free associations and were potentially amenable to introspection and therefore interpretation, these "hitherto unknown needs" had to be perceived by the analyst through empathic[2] recognition of the developmental meaning of the patient's unsymbolized behavior (since they weren't represented in any form within the patient's subjectivity), and addressed with non-interpretive methods such as assistance with tension regulation, tactful confrontation, various kinds of help with self-organization, and other forms of "psychological instruction" as needed.

While, because of its positivistic precision, I have never been able to use Gedo's specific 5-mode treatment model, I have found the general sensibility he was advocating, with its distinction between *phenomenologically experienced* and *objectively perceived* needs, to be essential to my understanding of different kinds of therapeutic-relational need. Like Gedo (to his credit), I believe that all patients manifest different levels of psychic functioning either simultaneously or oscillating over time; thus, most present with some unique combination of these two kinds of need. I credit Gedo with sensitizing me to the importance of objective needs and emboldening me to respond to such needs in ways that, prior to his contribution, would have seemed analytically unacceptable.

The essay that follows grows out of this sensibility. It deals with a particular application of this typology of needs: a proposed clinical theory and approach to patients presenting with serious self-care problems and lacunae, as these are perceived by the analytic therapist. However, the general model I develop here has potential applicability in a broad range of complex clinical situations. One example is situations in which the clinical couple is dealing explicitly with socio-political factors affecting the patient's self-care and/or well-being at the same time that they are working with the intrapsychic sequelae of early familial relational trauma. In a case reported by Rozmarin (2009) and discussed in IARPP Colloquium Series: No. 28 (2016), the analyst felt it necessary, at a critical juncture, to exhort the patient—an Israeli immigrant like himself—not to return to Israel to rejoin the army in order fight in a newly declared war against the Palestinians. The analyst did this because he believed strongly (in his heart) that the patient "needed" to hear this from him in service to both his physical and psychological well-being. The model developed here could help ground such interventions within a frame that retains its essential analytic properties.

The conundrum of self-care[3]

Self-care is a concept that has evocative meanings for most of us. Most of us, in one way or another, struggle to reconcile parts of ourselves that move in the direction of taking care of ourselves with those parts that move in directions we know to be deleterious to our well-being. I do not mean to imply that what constitutes taking care of oneself and what does not is always clear-cut. But often a person is aware of her or his chronic patterns of poor self-care, and it is these patterns and their analytic treatment that I focus on in this chapter.

It is surprising that the problem of self-care has not been more frequently and explicitly named or marked in our literature given the pervasiveness of self-care problems in what our patients talk to us about. Krystal (1988) and McDougall (2001) both have addressed the issue within the narrower topic of addictions. Certainly, aspects of self-care are inherent in any discussion of behavior disorders (Goldberg, 1999) and eating disorders (Kainer, 1999; Petrucelli & Stuart, 2001). It is also likely that the problems I think of as self-care problems others might subsume under "deeper," more fundamental problems such as an oedipal conflict, an ego deficit, a problem of self-cohesion, a problem of self-regulation, or a dissociative or vertical split in the ego or self. Without denying the utility of these other perspectives. I believe that the concept of self-care itself, as a rubric for considering a broad range of clinical phenomena, opens a space for clinically useful theorizing. Specifically, I suggest that the emergence of self-care problems in the analytic setting tends to provoke a particular kind of countertransference response and that the management of that response can be crucial to the establishment of an intersubjective process that is facilitative of the patient's developing enhanced capacities for self-care.

My thinking about self-care draws loosely upon models emerging from psychoanalytic infancy research regarding the development of the capacity for self-regulation (Beebe & Lachmann, 2002; Sander, 1995). For these researchers, developing competence in self-regulation depends on prior experience of competent interactive regulation within either the mother-infant or psychoanalytic dyad. The main argument in this chapter rests on a similar assumption: namely, developing competence in self-care requires prior experience of competent "interactive care." At the same time, I want to emphasize that I view self-care as a more complex and developmentally sophisticated set of capacities than self-regulation, although certainly self-regulatory skills are involved in self-care. While the principles emerging from mother-infant research have had enormous heuristic value in our coming to better understand the non-verbal, implicit dimensions of adult treatment, I think it is important to keep in mind that parent-child interactions *throughout* childhood and adolescence may inform us about other dimensions of the adult analytic encounter.

Concerned action and empathic recognition

Central to my thinking about self-care is a Winnicottian appreciation for the need to preserve certain paradoxical or dialectical tensions in both the parent-child and analytic relationships.[4] It seems to me that the development of the various capacities involved in self-care rests on the maintenance of *a dialectical tension that proceeds throughout a child's development between, on the one hand, all that parents do (and worry about) in the service of nurturing, protecting, assisting, guiding, and shaping a child in ways the parents consider to be in the child's best interest, and, on the other hand, all that parents do (or refrain from doing) by way of recognizing the child's unique self, ways of being, personal agency, and developmental trajectories*. Although as analysts we tend to emphasize, even idealize, the second of these impulses, realistically children could not grow into functioning adults without a familial matrix that includes both kinds of parental response. If one were to characterize the "action" of development through this particular psychoanalytic lens, one might say there is a necessary dialectical tension between *concerned action* and *empathic recognition*. Optimally, parents' inclinations to guide and shape their child become increasingly informed by and integrated with their empathic recognition of the child's unique personality, capabilities, and developmental needs. While few if any parents consistently live up to this ideal, in the families of patients with serious self-care issues, this fragile dialectic has collapsed in one way or another. Consequently, when such patients enter analytic treatment they often pose therapeutic conundrums that challenge the therapist to discover and then sustain some paradoxical or dialectical tension that is unique in each case but is often a variation of the central dialectical tension between concerned action and empathic recognition. The conundrum is often initiated when we become drawn in, more than would usually be the case, to trying to be helpful or protective by being directive, offering advice or guidance, or being confronting or challenging. In effect, the patient's poor self-care evokes a kind of parental response. In the part of our psychoanalytic superegos that remains grounded in its classical roots, such interventions or tendencies represent some combination of misguided therapeutic zeal and countertransference acting out in need of self-analysis and containment. In more contemporary versions of this classical stance such countertransference tendencies might be regarded as projectively or intersubjectively induced impulses that should not be acted upon but rather processed internally by the analyst until she can make use of them for purposes of greater empathic grasp and interpretation (Joseph, 1989; Ogden, 1994, 1997).

Yet, we also now have published accounts from the likes of Kohut, who famously reported his intervention with a patient who had sped recklessly in his car to get to his appointment, but arrived late because he had been stopped for speeding, then responded belligerently to the officer who up to that point had been inclined to let him off with a warning. After listening to the patient's "outpouring" about this and knowing about other such incidents in his past, Kohut said, "I am about to give you the deepest interpretation of the analysis so far: You are a complete idiot!" Later in the session Kohut reports saying to the patient that "we needed to understand what in his past . . . had made him so vulnerable and led him to respond as he did, but that first things came first: if he killed or injured himself in an accident, we certainly could not analyze his motivations" (1984, p. 74). Kohut's story is an extreme example of the kinds of participation or enactment these patients can evoke.

One might correctly point out that the two modes of parental or analytic responsiveness I am describing are not exactly, or at least necessarily, dialectical opposites but rather have considerable overlap. An analyst's impulse to forcefully intervene may be empathic to some unconscious or unformulated need in the patient, or to some "need" perceived by the analyst that is not part of the patient's subjective experience, conscious or unconscious—for example, the "need" for some form of protection or instruction (Gedo, 1979). Conversely, an analyst's impulse to remain silent or to non-directively explore the patient's current self-state represent, from a certain perspective, forms of concerned involvement. Despite this overlap, I feel the two terms describe a frequently encountered and potentially generative felt tension within the analyst between the impulse to explore and empathically understand the patient in a "disinterested" way (or, as Bion wrote, without "desire"), and the impulse to influence, protect or otherwise move the patient, driven by a compelling sense of concern.

Definition of self-care problems

Different analysts and therapists might use the term self-care differently. For some, it might have to include a physical or practical component as in taking care of one's health and safety, or exercising basic self-organizing capacities. For others, myself included, self-care is a broader concept that might also include taking care of oneself within a relationship or making choices that are likely to enhance one's overall sense of well-being in the long run. For purposes of the present discussion my focus will be on *any perceived self-care problem that evokes an impulse toward concerned involvement of some kind: that is, an impulse toward some protective or directive intervention on the patient's behalf. I include here any problem the therapist feels should evoke such a response but for some reason does not.* Of course, any such countertransference reaction is, at least to some extent, specific to the analyst, or, more accurately, to the intersubjective system co-created by the analyst and the patient. The analyst responds to the patient's self-care problems with her total psychology, including her own history and conflicts around self-care.

Treatment model: maintaining dialectical/paradoxical tension

My thinking about the treatment of self-care problems grows out of my belief that for many patients who struggle with self-care issues empathic understanding is necessary but not sufficient: They also, at times, require some form of concerned action. Kainer (1999), using language that is evocative of both Buddhist psychology (e.g., Nhat Hanh, 1998) and Fonagy et al.'s (2002) concept of mentalization, writes that patients with lapses in self-care selectively lack the capacity to be mindful of their inner states and behavior because of comparable early lapses in their parents' capacities to be consistently mindful of the child's mental states. I am suggesting that these patients evoke in us a kind of involved mindfulness of their various self-states, including their behavior and its potentially dangerous consequences, as a preliminary stage to their developing this capacity for themselves. The question thus becomes how to make use of these evoked countertransference states in ways that ultimately are most likely to facilitate better self-care in the context of a relationship that is experienced as sufficiently "new."

I would propose as a preliminary answer to this question that when an analytic therapist experiences countertransference pulls toward some form of active concerned involvement, the therapist regard such pulls as *the opening of a paradoxical or dialectical potential space in the transference-countertransference relationship that offers an opportunity to rework and heal earlier systemic breakdowns in the dialectic between concerned action and empathic recognition.* The implication, as Winnicott might say, is that the paradox or dialectic not be prematurely or unreflectively resolved either in the direction of active involvement or empathic recognition, one exclusive of the other, but rather that the tension between them be maintained as a generative framework or holding environment for negotiating new possibilities for integrating interactive care and self-care.

Central to the maintenance of these dialectical tensions are various paradoxes related to personal agency. Problems of self-care are almost by definition problems of agency. Patients cannot bring themselves to do that which they ostensibly want to do or feel they should do or should be able to do. One implication of my model is that the process of co-constructing the patient's sense of agency requires the therapist to hold in tension the following seemingly contradictory considerations: (1) her efforts to help the patient with self-care can only operate through the patient's agency—that is, the therapist cannot do anything "for" the patient; the patient must take it on as his own project; (2) the patient's sense of agency ultimately can only grow through a certain form of analytic unconditional acceptance and patience in conjunction with respect for the patient's autonomy; but

(3), paradoxically, the therapist (serving as the patient's "agent") must also be willing to assertively or protectively intervene at appropriate points of concern, knowing that such interventions may well run the risk of being either rejected or submissively accepted by the patient in the moment. This is to say, there may be no escaping an inherent "messiness" in the process of negotiating the nature of the analyst's involvement.

The problem of agency is further clarified by recognizing that for many patients with self-care issues there are at least two types of self-care that interact in complex and fluid ways. The first is the kind I have been referring to so far in this chapter. It is the form of self-care that most of us in contemporary Western middle and upper class culture strive for. In addition to the most basic self-care functions that might be assessed in a mental status evaluation, it includes such domains as health- and psychological health-fostering behaviors, various forms of self-organization and discipline, and behaviors conducive to professional, social and romantic success. At the "high" end one might include intellectual, cultural, ethical, and spiritual strivings, and virtually any form of practical knowledge or discipline pertaining to moving through life with greater success, enjoyment, fulfillment, and peace of mind.

The second form of self-care might be thought of as "compensatory self-care." These are the ways that we "take care of ourselves" that provide immediate pleasure, gratification, relief, solace or self-soothing—ways we have found to "reward" or regulate ourselves. Often we experience these forms of self-care as both compelling and shameful. Usually, if not always, these kinds of self-care seem to stand in direct opposition to and undermine the first kind. For example, an overweight patient revealed that she often longs for and rewards herself with a crème brûlée. By "taking care of herself" in one sense, she is specifically failing to do so in the other. Another patient who spends hours looking at pornography on the Internet rather than looking for a job is taking care of himself in one sense while failing to do so in another. Or a depressed patient who goes out drinking and doing socially "edgy" things with friends to compensate for what she feels is her boring, disappointing life, is taking care of herself in certain ways that work against taking care of herself in others.

One of the essential elements in helping our patients achieve greater capacities for self-care in the first sense is coming to a full recognition of the power of this second form of self-care as it operates in the patient's life.

(See S. Stern, 1992, for an earlier rendering of this therapeutic function.) Often, such forms of self-care represent ways the patient has developed to deal with the collapse of the dialectics of parental care described earlier. Close analysis may reveal an unconscious calculus, grounded in cynicism about the possibility of ever receiving real care from another person, wherein certain patients maintain a non-negotiable balance between what they experience themselves as giving and receiving within their intersubjective worlds. Here again, strengthening the patient's agency involves a paradox: The analyst tries to maintain a kind of equidistance (A. Freud, 1937) from the patient's conflicting self-care systems, seeking only empathic recognition, yet at the same time persists as a "quiet" advocate for the patient's movement toward better self-care.

The actual working out of the dialectical tensions I am describing can take many forms and is uniquely co-constructed by each analytic dyad. It may take the form of two different modes of intervention at different times, as in Kohut's example. But it may also take the form of an explicit negotiation of the therapist's role, or the development of a unique way of speaking, which somehow takes into account both poles of the dialectic. It seems to me, actually, that these characterizations are really only surface descriptions of an intersubjective process that is more fully captured by systems concepts such as Sander's (1995) notion of "system competence," Tronick's (1998) concept of "dyadic states of consciousness," and Benjamin's (2004) concept of the "intersubjective third." The yield of a successful struggle with the dialectic between concerned action and empathic recognition is that eventually the patient and therapist seem to enter an intersubjective space in which what the therapist thinks, feels, and says is received by the patient in a way that makes interactive care possible.

I do not want to give the impression that entire treatments are consumed with the kinds of management considerations I am outlining. These are analytic treatments first and foremost, and as such, proceed in an open-ended way, driven by the patient's concerns, self-presentation, and associations, and the analyst's spontaneous participation in response to the patient. The self-care problems emerge from this intersubjective interaction, and I am suggesting ways of thinking about how to respond when they do. These guidelines do not compel concerned action in all situations involving self-care problems. An analyst may well decide that the best "care" for a given patient is to remain in an empathic-exploratory-interpretive position.

The overweight patient who liked crème brûlée had a mother who had been narcissistically over-involved and over-invested in the patient's self-care efforts, especially in relation to eating and exercise. A previous therapist had made the mistake of trying to "work" with the patient around her moderate overeating—an involvement the patient ultimately experienced as a toxic repetition. While the patient understood that, in the long run, I wanted her to feel good about her eating and weight, we both understood that she could not tolerate my being invested in her undertaking any particular program in this or any other area of self-care. My genuine non-investment and patience in this sphere (i.e., my adherence to a disinterested, empathic-interpretive stance), and her gradual internalization of my attitude, contributed to her eventually being able to undertake a sustained weight-loss program. My point is not that the empathic-interpretive stance is never sufficient in self-care cases. It is that it is not sacrosanct and is more optimally understood as existing in dialectical tension with concerned action.

What makes the model analytic, moreover, is the analyst's commitment to subjecting any role-responsive enactments that occur to ongoing analytic reflection and, when appropriate, open dialogue. Gill (1994), Ehrenberg (1992), Ringstrom (1998), and Pizer (2004) all have stressed this point. Such dialogue is one of the elements that potentially establishes the analytic relationship as different from old toxic relationships. It also supports the patient's autonomy and agency by making explicit and demystifying the analyst's various kinds of participation.

I also do not want to give the impression that the dynamics around self-care all occur at a predominantly conscious level. Patients' problems with self-care are grounded in complex early relational histories, and these histories, like any patient's traumatic history, are bound to be unconsciously reenacted in the transference-countertransference relationship, even as the more conscious countertransference reactions I have described are emerging and being negotiated. For example, as part of such an enactment the analyst or therapist may find herself subjected to conditions in the transference-countertransference that undermine the therapist's ability to take care of herself in relation to the patient. Such an enactment may call for the therapist to take steps to establish a position of better self-care, and these actions may register with the patient in such a way as to affect the patient's own capacities for self-care. In this sense it is the analytic relationship as a whole that constitutes the total care system that ultimately impacts the patient's self-care capacities.

Clinical example: Mary

Mary was a chronically anorexic woman I saw in twice weekly analytic therapy. 5′5″ tall, Mary had maintained her weight at about 90 lb for many years. She appeared shockingly thin. While not exactly in denial about her eating disorder, Mary proceeded initially as if this were not a major concern. Her chief concern was that her two previous lengthy therapies had not helped her deal with her paralyzing self-criticalness—the legacy of her relationship with her toxically controlling and critical mother. The mother, who seemed to be very primitively organized, had treated Mary as a defective object whom she needed to constantly monitor and control. This included monitoring and regulating her eating and bowel functions. Mary had had to read her mother's mind and moods and accommodate her needs or face her angry, disapproving, guilt-inducing withdrawal. The result, Mary was aware, was that she had internalized her mother's critical voice.

What I wish to highlight is the particular way Mary and I worked out the balance between interactive and self-care within the context of the evolving transference-countertransference relationship. It was my assumption that her low weight was compromising her physical and psychological functioning, including her capacity to fully utilize therapeutic help. But it was not clear that the impairment was significant enough to warrant departing from my analytic approach in which the patient "guides" the process through her spontaneous self-presentation. I relied on my evolving countertransference responses to guide me on this question. Initially, I found myself content to wait for Mary to bring her anorexia into our dialogue. She seemed to have more pressing concerns, and I found these compelling and fully engaging.

One of her pressing concerns from the outset was her experience of me as someone to whom she looked for help moderating her paralyzingly self-critical, self-negating inner voice and the anxious-depressive self-states this voice constantly provoked. There was the sense of her being helpless to get out from under this oppressive introjected voice, and therefore of being dependent on my interventions to alleviate it. Thus, she constantly scanned and scrutinized my words and demeanor to see if I seemed to be feeling positively or negatively toward her. Silence and apparent emotional neutrality were experienced as implicit condemnation. And interpretations could easily be experienced as pathologizing criticisms. As part of this transference Mary sometimes sought explicit feedback about how I experienced her. I was willing on several occasions to reassure her that I felt warmly toward her and looked forward to our sessions. This feedback seemed to help her enormously in the short-run. However, as part of this same transference, she often experienced me as less warm and interactive than she would have liked. This caused her to question our fit, and wonder if she needed a different therapist. Yet, there was also a sense of a deepening bond between us, and a sense that our work together was addressing fundamental problems.

It was within this context that the conundrum of her poor self-care gradually presented itself. About one year into our treatment Mary went for a job interview and the HR interviewer asked her directly about her eating disorder and whether she would make sure to wear long sleeves and pants so as not to alarm the company's clients. Mary took offense at these intrusive questions but they shocked her out of her quasi-denial. She asked me how I had responded to her appearance when I first met her. I said that I had been shocked by it at first, but had gotten lulled into not focusing on it by our very engaging work together.

That experience marked a turning point in our treatment. For the first time I became more confronting, and Mary became more receptive regarding the intractability of her anorexia. I said that maybe this experience shocked us both into realizing we needed to take this more seriously. She became extremely anxious and asked if I thought her gaining weight was necessary for her to get better. I was able to say with conviction that I absolutely thought so, that I was sure her restrictive eating was masking important anxieties and emotions, and that I thought that if she was not able to eat and gain weight, this would limit how much the therapy would ultimately help her. Mary was obviously both frightened and relieved to hear me say this. At some level she knew I was right, but the prospect of gaining weight terrified her.

It was at this point that, for the first time, we began discussing how we should together approach her eating and weight gain. I was aware of the enormous risk that she might experience me as monitoring and evaluating her progress, thereby malignantly repeating her mother's critical over-involvement. I suggested she begin keeping a log of her daily food intake and that after a week or so I would show it to a nutritionist who was very knowledgeable about anorexia. She agreed, and conscientiously complied. The nutritionist became an important symbolic figure in the background. She read Mary's logs and sent them back with written feedback in the margins. She complimented Mary on what she was doing well, and made sensitively worded suggestions about what needed to change: most importantly, she needed to increase her calories until she started gaining weight.

Mary tried at first to make her own bargain with these suggestions, for example, by setting arbitrary daily calorie goals. She would bring in her logs and show me the changes she was making, and the days she was and wasn't meeting her goals. This was a critical point in our negotiation of my role. How involved should I become here? Should I compliment her when she met her goals? How should I respond when she did not? Should I question her about weight gain? It seemed that for a while our focus on her eating was taking up most of our time, leaving little room for the pressing emotional concerns that had occupied us until now. I found myself drifting into the role of policeman, as if it were my job to make sure she was not fooling herself and actually gaining weight. Imperceptibly, our alliance started to erode. She clearly was more anxious during her sessions, and became resistant to talking about her eating. I picked up on this and wondered out loud what was happening. Mary wasn't sure, although she agreed that something had changed between us. I said I was worried that we had lost something that we had had in the process of working on her eating. I affirmed that our relationship was the most important thing, and that the eating program could not be allowed to threaten that. But, then, what should my role be?

This is precisely the kind of therapeutic conundrum that my model speaks to. The time had clearly arrived when I felt an impulse toward more concerned involvement, but the question was: what sort of involvement? As I have argued, optimally this situation sets in motion a dialectical process wherein the balance between concerned action and empathic recognition becomes the focus of ongoing negotiation.

With Mary, what we arrived at was that my job was to represent reality and perhaps nudge her in what I felt was a healthy direction, but not to police her eating. Reality, as I saw it, included the following: First and foremost, she, not I, needed to be responsible for her eating. I could register my concern, but not be an enforcer. Second, if she wanted to gain weight, she would have to increase her calories until she actually gained weight. Third, if she did gain weight it would undoubtedly be very frightening and difficult, but I would be there for her as it happened. As I stated earlier, any surface characterization of this kind of negotiation does not do justice to the deeper intersubjective processes that take place. In Mary's case, the "stance" I have described was the surface resolution of this kind of intersubjective merger. Out of our particular dialectical process Mary gradually took on the weight gain project as her own, and became determined not to let either physical or psychological obstacles deter her for long. She began to increase her calories in a more determined way, and she began to gain weight. Pound by pound she moved up, hitting her first wall at 95, working through it, reaching 100, hitting the next wall which lasted well over a year, and then gaining to 105. Interestingly, as she assumed the responsibility for her weight gain it occupied less of our time in sessions, though we needed periodically to return to her eating, each time reworking exactly where I positioned myself in relation to it. Over time Mary's eating became less of a struggle, she made difficult adjustments to changes in her body (which fortunately she was able to discuss with me in graphic detail), and her weight gain was clearly associated with a greater sense of substantiality and aliveness.

As mentioned earlier, the interactions around self-care do not all occur at the conscious level but often enter the transference-countertransference relationship unconsciously through enactments that repeat the conditions of the patient's childhood. Such an enactment occurred between Mary and me sometime during the first year of our co-created eating program.

For reasons that even now remain obscure, Mary entered a months-long period when she was having apparently grave doubts about her treatment with me. She was anxious and self-conscious during our sessions, often saying that she didn't know what to talk about, even though there were things that had occurred to her during the week, between sessions. She also wasn't talking about her eating, and she didn't look good. She couldn't put her finger on what was wrong except that she felt she needed something more or different from me than she was getting. She knew and appreciated that I listened attentively, and knew that my open-ended approach had helped us discover many things about her that we otherwise might not have.

But the problem, I knew, was that she had such a powerful internalized critical voice that she needed almost constant reassurance from me to counteract it. Even though I did feel very positively toward her, and on occasion authentically offered her such reassurance, it was not my style to do this all the time; nor did I feel, at some level, that this was all that Mary needed. I sensed it might be important to stay with her frustration.

As her frustration mounted she again brought up her thoughts about possibly seeing a different therapist, although she did so reluctantly since she worried that she might hurt my feelings to the point I would want to be rid of her. While I did not want to be rid of her, I did start to wonder if perhaps she was right: maybe a warmer more active therapist would be better. In one session I shared these questions, and Mary became terrified. The next session she came back after being acutely anxious and depressed since our previous session, worried that I was losing faith in her therapy. This reassured me that what was happening was more of a transference-countertransference enactment than a literal questioning of the therapy on Mary's part. I assured her I was still very committed to continuing our work.

But her expressed frustration did not abate, and there was the persistent feeling that she was not getting what she needed. At this point I was questioning my ability to treat Mary, and beginning to feel badly about myself for not being warmer and more interactive: Why couldn't I just be the kind of therapist she needed me to be? I worried: was she destined to repeat another failed therapy? Then slowly, it began to dawn on me that we were reenacting Mary's relationship with her mother, and I was in Mary's position. She had me doubting my very competence as a therapist and person, wishing I were someone I wasn't, and feeling very anxious about failing to meet her needs. This realization emboldened me. When Mary next voiced her frustrations, I finally said that I thought I was feeling something like what she used to feel with her mother. I felt as if she needed me to be someone I wasn't, and it had me feeling badly about myself as a therapist. I said I could only be who I was, that I had my strengths and limitations, and that we had somehow to face that together. I said I felt very confident of my positive feelings toward her, and was sorry she could not experience them more. I would try to express them more freely, but there was probably a limit to how much I could comfortably do this. As I said all this, I felt a combination of relief and grief, as if I, or we together, were beginning to face a painful loss. Mary, though not able to say much in response at the time, was clearly surprised and moved by this pronouncement. She has, subsequently, been able to articulate how powerfully my openness during this session affected her.

This intervention had a profound impact on both of us. It cured me of my anxiety about disappointing her, and somehow it helped Mary move past her apprehensions about me, and our work together. One could speculate about the therapeutic action of this intervention. What seems clearest to me is that, in standing up for my own personhood—*a form of self-care within the countertransference*—I ceased being an "old object" and became a kind of "new object" for Mary, although not exactly the new object that she had been hoping for. I was not the new object who gave her everything she needed, but a new object who balanced giving her some of what she needed and not losing myself in the process.

This kind of expressive intervention and interpretation of a reenactment is not, at this point, a novel analytic technique. Such interventions virtually define the contemporary Relational-psychoanalytic contribution to the theory of technique and therapeutic action. All I am adding to what we already understand about such interventions is that they represent, in certain instances, a form of analytic self-care that emerges within the transference-countertransference relationship. Even this understanding is implicit in the work of Weiss and Sampson (1986), Bollas (1987), and Ehrenberg (1992). Yet, I feel it takes on an added dimension of meaning when examined within the context of a theory of self-care.

Conclusion: the model's larger utility

I conclude this chapter with the suggestion that the principles I have been outlining have potentially very broad applicability within many analytic treatments. While serious self-care problems bring these principles into sharp relief, I believe that in fact we often find ourselves struggling between impulses to assist or exhort our patients in one way or another, and disciplining ourselves to simply "stay with" the patient's subjective experience as the basis for ever-deepening analytic empathy and understanding. I believe the model I have proposed offers a useful way to think about this kind of conundrum: one that confers legitimacy upon, and offers the possibility of integrating, both sides of the technical dilemma in a way that is therapeutically more powerful than opting unquestioningly to resolve the struggle in one direction or the other.

Notes

1 As a clarifying analogy, think of the difference between a young child's *felt* need for attention or mirroring attunement and that same child's "need" to have caregivers prevent them from running out into busy streets, or "need" to be assisted in learning essential developmental skills of all kinds, ranging from toilet training to language acquisition to social, psychological, organizational, and self-care skills—that is, needs that are not subjectively experienced but rather must be *perceived* by caregiving others responsible for a child's care and socialization.

2 Gedo's usage of the word empathy here was closer to Winnicott's (1960a) characterization of a good-enough mother's attunement to the needs of her preverbal baby than to Kohut's (e.g., 1982, 1984) "empathic attunement" with a patient's subjective experience, which, as I read him, could include either states within or outside reflective awareness.

3 Originally published in *Contemporary Psychoanalysis*, *43*: 605–620 (2007).

4 While my thinking in this chapter is most directly influenced by Winnicott, I am aware that the relational sensibility with which I approach the issues owes much to the work of Hoffman (1998) and Pizer (1998), both of whom have shaped contemporary thinking about the omnipresence of paradox, dialectical tension, negotiation, and choice in the analytic process.

Chapter 8

Analytic peace

In a recent session with Suzanne, after listening to her scattered narrative for half an hour, I had the thought, and said to her, that I heard two main themes embedded in what she was talking about: contentment and longing. This interested her. I said further that, at least at the moment, her feelings of contentment seemed to be mainly in relation to me, and her feelings of longing seemed directed mainly toward her mother. She smiled at feeling recognized, yet the smile itself struck me as expressing the very tension I had just named. She was at once pleased and calmed by this further evidence that I was doing my job well (a concern of hers in the analysis as elsewhere in her life), but my calling attention to her longing prompted a more conscious, and thus more painful, awareness of it. "Why do I *do* that?" she asked in a pleading tone that conveyed desperation, self-recrimination, and a hint of ironic pleasure that things weren't as bad as they used to be. Our attempt to answer this question together organized our dialogue for the duration of the session.

Taking my characterization of this session as a microcosm, most psychoanalytic papers focus on the second part of Suzanne's current experience: her painful internal struggle with her mother and the implied analytic work that still lies ahead. In this final chapter I wish to focus on the first part: the sense of contentment in relation to me that Suzanne was experiencing as the result of work already done. This session occurred approximately one year following the crisis in Suzanne's treatment described in Chapter 2, the resolution of which had had such a transformative effect. The relative calm and contentment in Suzanne's voice a year later still embodies this transformation.

* * *

Freud (1912a, 1912b, 1913, 1914, 1915a) often characterized the analytic process as a kind of battle—a battle between the analyst and the patient's resistances, and between the patient and his own resistances. While it is true we have moved away from this adversarial sensibility, it is also true that our patients are still engaged in battles. Now, however, the nature and locus of the battles has shifted. We now understand that our patients struggle for psychic survival against powerfully destructive forces that exist in the intermediate area between past and present, outside and inside, other and self. This is not the creative intermediate area of Winnicott's (1971a) transitional and cultural phenomena but its malignant twin wherein the effects of childhood traumatic experience come to occupy, and repeat themselves endlessly within, each patient's subjective and intersubjective worlds. Consequently, much of our contemporary psychoanalytic literature still reads like a therapeutic war room. It gives us powerful theories and tools for dealing with impasses, enactments, doer/done-to complementarities (Benjamin, 2004), subjugating thirds (Ogden, 1994), psychic deadness (Eigen, 1996; Ogden, 1997), and destructiveness that must be survived (Winnicott, 1971a; Benjamin, 1990). This is as it should be. Given the nature of our patients' battles as we now understand them, we know that we will be drawn into their malignant intermediate zones with them, that their struggles must be engaged in some form within the transference-countertransference relationship if real analytic transformation—transformation "from the inside out" (Bromberg, 1991; Mitchell, 1997, p. 52)—is to occur.

All of this is a given in what follows. However, in this chapter I want to come at it from the other side. Instead of focusing on the nature of the patient's struggles, and those that come to occupy the analytic dyad, I wish instead to focus on the nature of the analytic experience that marks the resolution and transformation of the intersubjective struggles of the analytic dyad, and ultimately the intrapsychic struggles of the patient. Of course, it is true that every patient's, and every analytic dyad's, struggles are unique; thus the therapeutic transformations or resolutions of those struggles are also unique in each case, reflecting the particularities of the patient's old object relationships and trauma history, the complexities of the patient's psychological organization, and the unique qualities of the new relational experience with the analyst. At the same time, I want to assert that there is a universal, or nearly universal, aspect to the resolution of all analytic struggles: the experience of a state I would describe as *analytic peace.* I have become increasingly convinced of its universality because, since formulating the concept, I now hear patients (such as Suzanne) referring or implicitly alluding to it more often, either as a felt experience in the here-and-now or as a longed-for state that would represent deliverance from their particular pain or struggles. Indeed, the idea first came to me when two patients on the same day made direct reference to peaceful states experienced during a session (see below).

The concept is especially appealing to me because there are continuities between analytic peace and forms of peace achieved in other life domains such as the political and spiritual. Peace always exists in relation to struggle, tension, or conflict, and acquires its meaningfulness as an emergence from, or mastery of, these painful states. The achievement of peace is such a universally desirable experience—indeed, one of the core values or goals implicit in being human—that identifying it as central to the psychoanalytic enterprise underlines the fact that psychoanalysis deals in similarly universal human struggles. At the same time, what interests me about the concept is that the state of peace achieved in an analytic relationship has unique characteristics specific to that context. Thus, while a sometime-meditator myself, and thus respectful of contemporary approaches that seek to integrate meditation practice or mindfulness training and psychotherapy, I believe that psychoanalytic therapy yields its own forms of peace as a function of the analytic process itself and the specifically analytic forms of wisdom guiding that process.

There are theoretical precursors to the experience I am identifying. Within classical psychoanalysis and ego psychology, the experience of *safety*, as described for example by Sandler (1960), Schafer (1983), and Weiss, Sampson et al. (1986), is one such concept. Another is Sullivan's (1953) concept of *security*, which he essentially defined as the absence of interpersonal anxiety. Kohut's (1971, 1977) *selfobject experience*, especially idealizing selfobject experience in which a sense of calm results from a felt merger with the idealized parent/analyst, informs my understanding of analytic peace. Winnicott's (1960a) *holding* moves in a similar direction. With reference to holding, Winnicott wrote: "This essential maternal function enables the mother to know about her infant's earliest expectations and needs, and makes her personally satisfied in so far as the infant *is at ease*" (1960a, p. 148, emphasis added).

Bion's (1962) *container/contained* paradigm refers essentially to a peace-engendering function of both mother and analyst. Through the mother/analyst's reverie capacities the infant/patient's overwhelming (and therefore projected) affects are processed in such a way as to make them less anxiety-provoking and more tolerable. Indeed, the implication of Bion's formulations is that *thinking* itself, especially thinking about one's most disturbing emotional experience, requires a certain level of calm relative to those emotions—calm that has been intersubjectively achieved. Finally, some research-based concepts—Bowlby's (1975, 1988) *secure attachment*, Beebe and Lachmann's (2002, 2014) *interactive regulation*, and Schore's (1994, 2003) *affect regulation*—overlap with my ideas about analytic peace. The universality of these various peace-like concepts suggests that the achievement of a sense of peace in analysis is one of its deeply implicit aims.

Analytic peace, as I define it, is a mental state (relief, relaxation, calm, contentment,) that emerges from another mental state (tension, conflict, anxiety, worry, torment, pain) as a result of analytic work—work that is simultaneously intersubjective and intrapsychic. The concept of analytic peace is elusive and saturated with paradoxical and dialectical tensions, some of which will be discussed in later sections. Peace is never completely or finally achieved, in analysis or in life: Finding a sense of inner peace is a life-long struggle for most of us. Moreover, its achievement in analysis is always relative—a step or transformative moment in the cumulative process of emergence *from* each patient's (and each dyad's) particular struggles and *toward* an increasingly resilient sense of peace relative to those struggles.

I view the achievement of a sense of relative peace as a transcendent analytic aim because it is an encompassing mental state that registers the condition of the patient's psyche (conscious and unconscious; symbolized and unsymbolized) in a given moment relative to his struggles and therefore relative to the core implicit aims of the treatment. Among the superordinate aims of analysis that have been written about, the sense of peace seems to me on a par with, and related to, the sense of *aliveness* (Winnicott, 1971a; Ehrenberg, 1992; Eigen, 1996; Ogden, 1997). Similar to peace, aliveness is an encompassing subjective state that registers the condition of the patient's (and/or analyst's) psyche in the moment relative to a core dimension of many patients' struggles:

a sense of psychic deadness or feeling of being less than human. Although, within the peculiar legacy of classical psychoanalytic metapsychology, peace and aliveness might seem to be opposite states (eros vs. thanatos), most contemporary analysts would, on reflection, recognize that they are complexly interconnected: *Feeling more alive makes one feel more at peace, and feeling more peaceful makes it possible to live more fully.* Winnicott famously implored: "May I be alive when I die" (C. Winnicott, 1978, quoted in Eigen, 1996). I suspect most of us would concur but would add that we also hope to feel at peace, whatever that might mean for each of us.

Peace as an intersubjective achievement

Common to all of the predecessor concepts reviewed above is the, perhaps obvious, understanding that a patient's achievement of a state of peace in an analytic context is always, first, a two-person, intersubjective achievement. Something must happen between the patient and analyst (meaning, usually, many things over a long period of time) that transforms the patient's state of tension or struggle into a different state characterized by greater calm and relief from struggle. Note that by "intersubjective achievement" I don't necessarily imply that the therapist always experiences a state of peacefulness along with the patient, although this certainly can and does happen. The analyst brings complex (conscious and unconscious) processing and relational capacities to the analytic encounter part of whose reason for being is to engage the patient in ways that ultimately yield experiences of greater peace relative to his struggles. These processing and relational capacities amount to a hard-won and specifically analytic form of wisdom that the analyst hopefully has cultivated through immersion in analytic work and ideas, and a capacity to "learn from experience" (Bion, 1962) as a product of that immersion. Thus, in a general way one might say that analytic peace typically begins as a complex state or potential "in" the analyst. But it is hardly the case that the analyst always feels peaceful, or even, necessarily, feels peaceful concurrently with the patient's reaching that state. In short, what I mean by the statement that peace must begin as an intersubjective achievement is that the patient can, at first, only experience peace relative to his core struggles in the context of intersubjective experiences with the analyst *of one kind or another* that somehow produce such feelings *in the patient.*

Necessity, tension, and peace

In the final paragraphs of Chapter 4, in the context of proposing a *principle of necessity* as an unseen driver of the analytic process, I suggested: (1) that the principle of necessity expresses itself as felt tensions within the analytic field related to the patient's struggles; and (2) that the waning of these tensions as a result of successful analytic work is synonymous with the emergence of a felt sense of peace relative to those tensions and struggles. I likened the intersubjective achievement of states of analytic peace to the calm that overtook the infant daughter in Sander's video clip (see Chapter 1, p. 00) as her hand grasped her father's finger and she fell asleep. Given the nature of many of our patients' trauma histories, however, any such movement toward relaxation and peace also may signify increased vulnerability and thus immediately call into play paranoid-schizoid defenses (self-protective operations; repetitive transferences)—that is, new tensions that now occupy center stage and must be met in new ways necessitated by each new iteration of the patient's struggles and those of the dyad.

The relationship I am theorizing between these three phenomena—(1) the principle of necessity, (2) the felt tensions "produced" by necessity, which come to occupy and structure the analytic field, and (3) emergent experiences of peace relative to these tensions—has clinical utility, but only in a complex, indirect way. I began this book cautioning against the problem of *confusing the means with the end*: the error that occurs when "the goal of offering patients the unique forms of help they need to achieve their own therapeutic objectives can subtly shift to helping them attain an ideal end state envisioned by the analyst's theory." While the arrival of states of analytic peace *is* a desired end state, there is no clearly delineated theoretical/technical path toward achieving it. For the most part, it is not a state that an analytic therapist aims directly to produce. The particular contours of what constitutes analytic peace, and how it is achieved, are unique for each patient and dyad, and its arrival is unpredictable and emergent from the process of helping the patient with his struggles via the co-creation and evolution of the complex needed analytic relationship.

Analysis by definition entails the invitation and opening up of struggle, a *moving into* what has previously been intolerable: at worst, a combination of catastrophic anxiety, unbearable emotional pain, and psychic chaos or fragmentation. The fact that this moving into the intolerable can *only* occur *intersubjectively* due to the psychological impossibility of experiencing such unbearable states in isolation is one of the fundamental realities that make psychoanalysis necessary (Poland, 2000). The analyst's capacity to accompany the patient into this experience of the intolerable, and the patient's progressive willingness to grant the analyst entry into his most vulnerable, guilt-and-shame-filled areas of trauma, are some of the major elements that hold the possibility and hope of transforming struggle into peace, and that distinguish the peace achieved through analysis from that achieved in other life domains and practices.

Thus striving (in too direct a way) to relieve patients of their struggles usually works against accomplishing that; whereas "staying with" the struggle, seeking to discern all of its elements (conscious and unconscious), witnessing it (Poland, 2000; Reis, 2009; Gerson, 2009), processing it internally and intersubjectively over time, finding ways of meeting the struggle through some deeply felt communication with oneself or the patient (Bollas, 1987), even, in certain cases, sharing in the despair of never seeming to find relief (Winnicott, 1960b; Gerson, 2009; M. Slavin, 2010), tend to be what is actually helpful. One might summarize the paradoxes here by saying that analytic peace is not pursued as a therapeutic "desire" in the Bionian sense; rather it exists as a *beacon* toward which one orients and moves, but always via unknown, unpredictable pathways of struggle, inquiry, and co-creativity.

At the same time, paradoxically, having peace in mind as a superordinate aim of analysis opens up one's thinking about therapeutic possibilities in new ways. As one gets deeply into an analytic relationship, unique interventions and interactions emerge that specifically address the patient's core struggles in complex but powerful ways, including interventions that do not fall within existing categories of therapeutic action or therapist participation. For example, I have found that with certain patients something one might call an "analytic mantra" emerges, which comes to have particular force or leverage as it is repeated selectively during a period of the treatment.

Clint

I think here of Clint, a patient in late middle age who tended to speak in articulate but very general ways about what he wanted in his life but had never achieved, and about his negative expectancies about what was possible for him in the future. It was easy for me to get almost hypnotically lulled into Clint's pessimism because of his lyrical eloquence, and because the evidence of his life accomplishments up until the present seemed to support his gloomy predictions. He had failed in certain ways—failures that were understandable in light of his powerful, sadistic father's systematic efforts to undermine and crush his sense of competence and potency as an adolescent and young adult. Finally, at some point it dawned on me that, while Clint's narrative had some basis in reality, he was in fact telling himself a story—a version of the story his father had told him about himself. From this point on I began saying in a playful but serious way: *"I don't trust any generalizations you make about yourself or your future. I think we do better to stay with what is happening, and what you're feeling, now."* This became a kind of mantra for us for quite a while: one that always brought a knowing smile and a palpable sense of relief—relief that grew over time. It became part of the bulwark we were gradually constructing against the crushing power of the internalized voice of his father, and a marker of the potential space we were co-creating for the emergence of a new sense of self grounded in his own deeper belief about what was possible for him in what remained of his life. Of course, the mantra derived its power not only from its content but from its tone (knowing, playful, affectionate, supportive) and the fact that it came from me—a new kind of male authority figure who saw both Clint's potential and the forces he was battling in his efforts to actualize it.

One characteristic of my intervention with Clint was that it was at once both an "objective" and "subjective" statement. That is, it was both a kind of interpretation naming an emotional, intrapsychic truth I had identified, *and* a complexly caring and supportive statement the intention of which was to counteract (and help him counteract) destructive patterns of thought that were interfering with his movement toward greater self-confidence, agency, and ultimately, peace (Sander's *specificity of recognition* and *specificity of connection*). As I have said repeatedly in earlier chapters, I regard this fusion of truth-seeking and subjective engagement in the analyst's language and voice as central to the analyst's holding function. The particular fusion and quality of objective and subjective elements evolve uniquely in every case and are part of the progressive fittedness that leads to greater system competence (Sander, 1995), and thus the potential for experiences of analytic peace. Over time this mixture of objectivity and subjectivity produces a knowing quality in the analyst's voice, which takes on soothing, peace-engendering properties for the patient. This form of knowing does not have as its complement the feeling of being objectified but rather the feeling of being known (Sander, 1995). Importantly, this knowing quality always exists in tension with the analyst's ceaseless openness to the surprising and not yet known or understood (Bion, 1970; D.B. Stern, 1990). The patient needs both conviction and uncertainty from the analyst (Hoffman, 1998): It is the combination that contributes to the holding environment that gradually and progressively put's the patient, in Winnicott's (1960a) words, "at ease."

Peace as the yield of working through

Another way of conceptualizing the existential relationship between the principle of necessity, the tensions that come to occupy the analytic field, and the emergence of analytic peace relative to the patient's struggles is as a framework for re-imagining Freud's (1914) concept of *working through.* In this frame, the achievement of states of relative peace become the *telos* of the working through process (see also Alizade, 2010).

The arrival of analytic peace is always unpredictable, complex, and emergent, but, as I began to suggest in the closing paragraphs of Chapter 4, often results from a working through of some core tension that has come to occupy the analysis. In contrast to Freud's formulation that what is worked through are resistances residing entirely within the patient, contemporary theories envision a process that is simultaneously *intersubjective and intrapsychic.* Moreover, whereas Freud's working through referred to a repetitive working over relatively fixed intrapsychic configurations (defenses against instinctual strivings), working through in this contemporary model is a moving target in which the complex effects of the patient's past are constantly reconfigured in the present interaction with the analyst such that the dyad is always co-creating anew that which is being worked on and worked through.

Finally, as in traditional theory, working through occurs for the most part incrementally, but it is the system as well as the individual patient that is undergoing incremental change. The analyst and patient live through things together, and *together* develop understandings (both explicit and implicit) and find ways of being with and speaking to each other that address the current struggle. Once a given tension is worked through, or partially worked through, the gain in system competence becomes a kind of way station or building block. In time, this sense of achievement will be lost as the patient's struggles find new ways of attaching and asserting themselves within the unpredictable, messy, and mostly unconscious happenings of the intersubjective encounter as it evolves, opening up new opportunities for working through. Working through, in this sense, refers to a non-linear process through which the system is continually morphing into new patterns of organization, but patterns that are increasingly more powerful in their capacity to help the patient with his struggles and achieve more reliable and sustainable experiences of analytic peace.

I say "for the most part incrementally" because, while incremental change creates a necessary backdrop, more dramatic changes can occur suddenly and unpredictably, either: (1) because of happenings in the patient's life; (2) through unpredictable interactions between the patient-analyst system and the outside (extra-analytic) world; or (3) through occurrences within the system (an empathic failure or precipitous enactment on the "negative" side, or, on the "positive" side, a new significant understanding, corrective relational experience, or breakthrough in a prolonged enactment).

Alan

To illustrate the relationship between incremental and more dramatic forms of working through, I offer the following highly condensed account of the evolution of the transference during my 10-year, twice-a-week treatment of Alan, a very bright, professionally successful, gay man who began treatment in his mid-30s. Given his history of feeling no one really understood or was there for him emotionally as a child—a feeling intensified by a severe learning disability and his confusion regarding his sexuality—Alan's primary transference anxiety took the form of having no faith that in a time of crisis I would really be there for him: My "caring" was strictly at a professional level. There was an easy rapport between us, and a generally positive transference with both mirroring and idealizing elements that developed as he gained confidence that I was capable of understanding and perhaps helping him. But he felt certain that there was a limit to my concern. He frequently referred to the case of a friend who had been in treatment with a local analyst. At her most depressed point the therapist had not made himself available, and she had committed suicide. Alan was generally skeptical of the medical and helping professions, assuming we were all basically in it for the money.

Sometime during the second year of therapy, Alan started calling between sessions when events in his life precipitated overwhelmingly anxious-depressed states. His attitude when he called was apologetic, not entitled. He would quickly get to the point, expressing directly the intensity of his affective state, and his helplessness at not knowing what to do about it. The average call lasted 10–15 minutes, and consisted mostly of my listening to him and then giving him some reality-based feedback or reassurance to offset his usually irrational, catastrophic fears. For example, if, as was often the case, Alan's crisis of the moment concerned some business setback that he believed threatened his entire career and future, I might say something like: "In all the time we have been meeting I have never known you *not* to be able to solve a business problem!" I could say this confidently because of Alan's complete brilliance in his particular line of work, evident even in the early stages of his career during which these crises occurred. At some point he would say: "OK, thanks Steve. That helps. I feel a little better. I'll see you Tuesday."

I believe Alan felt reasonably well understood, connected, and cared about from our work in sessions. There was a comfortable rhythm to our work, and an ease of affective communication. Undoubtedly, this work was gradually accruing toward a strengthened sense of self. But the work in sessions did not calm him when he was in one of his anxious-depressed states. My genuine (non-resentful) willingness to talk to him when he needed me, and the ritual we co-created during these calls, did have a calming effect, and over time the intensity of these states diminished, and his ability to manage them on his own improved.

During the late phase of therapy when, overall, Alan was feeling much more self-confident and self-reliant, he found himself in a major relationship crisis. The abandonment aspects of this crisis again precipitated his overwhelmed anxious-depressed states and again required between-session support, including some calls when I was on vacation, which Alan clearly appreciated. But the incident that convinced him beyond any further doubt of the genuineness of my caring for him, our most significant moment of meeting, was, ironically, one in which I was not directly involved at all. One evening during the crisis he called my home when I was not there. (This was before the era of cell phones.) Over the years he had called enough that my wife knew who he was, and they had spoken briefly on several occasions. I should say that Alan is an extremely warm, outgoing, even mildly exhibitionistic man; thus this very circumscribed telephone relationship that he cultivated with my wife was comfortable for him, and really for all three of us. During this particular call something about my wife's attunement to his sense of urgency, and reassurance that I would be home soon, led Alan to conclude that I had spoken to her about his crisis in a sympathetic rather than irritated way. For Alan, this was more compelling proof of my genuinely caring attitude than anything I had ever said to him directly. It was as if he now had closure on a question that had haunted him throughout all the previous years of treatment. And with this closure, and the deep sense of calm and confidence that accompanied it, he now had what he needed from me in order to move forward on his own. (Think again of the baby girl in Sander's video clip grasping her father's finger and falling asleep.) Termination occurred within a few months. Through periodic contacts he has initiated during the decade and a half since we ended, I know that this basic confidence and ability to regulate his own anxieties has held up well over time.

Working through, mourning, and peace

Working through means something different for every patient; yet there are certain components that seem nearly universal. One that has occupied a central place in psychoanalytic thinking from the beginning (Freud, 1917) is the *mourning process* involved in coming to terms with losses of all kinds, including the loss of that which one has never had. This is a large topic, especially in light of the problem that real grieving can only occur if there is a capacity to grieve, which in the case of the severely traumatized, or those operating primarily in a mode that is developmentally prior to Klein's (1946) "depressive position," may be compromised in profound and complex ways (S. Stern, 2015). The psychological configurations that stand in the way of being able to grieve almost by definition involve a deep sense of aloneness that must somehow be breached within the transference-countertransference relationship if the necessary grieving, and hence working through, is to become possible. Thus, with Alan, his progressive connection with and trust in me was accompanied by a gradual coming to terms with his aloneness as a child and the reasons for that aloneness, often marked by extreme sadness and sobbing. This progressive capacity to grieve, and the feeling of affective aliveness and integration that accompanies it, are central to the working through process and hence to the achievement of states of relative peacefulness. I regard Alan as a relatively "simple" case in this regard; for others more severely traumatized, such as Mary (see below), things tend to unfold in more tortuous and torturous ways.

* * *

In concluding this section there is an important caveat regarding the use of newly achieved states of relative peace as a criterion for a successful working through process: namely, the problem of knowing what is collusion or illusion vs. true peace. What feels like peace may, in fact, be a defensive avoidance of one or more forms of struggle. Of course, it may also be both.

Elizabeth

Elizabeth, a patient I saw for many years beginning when she was 18, had been severely sexually and emotionally abused throughout her late childhood and adolescence, and was hospitalized 5 times during the first 10 years of our work. Gradually, she came to experience me as a safe male figure who understood her struggles and accepted her as no one in her past ever had. The sense of safety had a literal quality: It was as if being under my care literally shielded her from the (now-unrealistic) threat she still experienced in relation to her early abusers. This sense of calm or safety came to be a central dimension of our relationship, and undoubtedly contributed to her growing resilience and strength over many years as this intersubjective state became increasingly consolidated. However, it gradually came to light that this state also was functioning dissociatively as a kind of refuge that was masking important, destabilizing aspects of her trauma history that were not sufficiently worked through, thus leaving her vulnerable to a kind of decompensation whenever something triggered traumatic emotional memories, flashbacks, and dreams. This realization (and interpretation) allowed her to confront these memories more intentionally, but now with the courage gained from years of "living" in the shared, relatively peaceful, space we had co-created in our relationship. After several additional years of working in this more courageous mode, Elizabeth achieved a more in-depth sense of peace, which she characterized as: "no longer feeling like a panicky 14-year-old for hours on end after I have a bad dream or memory. I feel like an adult."

This case example demonstrates, and helps to flesh out, a "peace sensibility" in two ways. First, in certain treatments it can happen that over time just being in the analyst's presence, and under the analyst's care, can come to have deeply peace-engendering qualities for the patient, which cumulatively foster development of the patient's capacity to experience states of peace on his own. Second, operating from this sensibility can at times involve confrontation—confrontation of the defensive, self-regulating, or more general characterological patterns that stand in the way of developing a deeper, more resilient sense of peace.

Close process illustrations

I mentioned at the beginning of this chapter that my initial formulation of the idea of analytic peace grew out of my work with two patients—specifically, two sessions on the same day in which both patients referred to peaceful feelings they were either having with me during the present session or had had in a previous session. Because I wanted to record something of the process that led me to conceive the idea, I jotted down notes from these sessions later in the day. I will share those notes verbatim (transcribed in italics), introducing them with some necessary background, and annotating them with interpolated comments set off in brackets.

A significant background factor in both cases was the unusual frame of the work. I moved to Portland, Maine, in 2003 after practicing for 20 years in Chicago. As part of my decision to move, I planned to continue my Chicago practice *in person* for at least a year following the move, requiring me to commute back and forth weekly and live essentially half-time in Chicago. As it turned out, I continued this *weekly* commute for two years. During that time I went through a process with every patient, exploring what each would do when I finally was no longer commuting. Where appropriate, I offered patients the opportunity to continue with me by phone. Then, as the time approached, I reached a new decision to continue commuting *one weekend a month* in order to see in person anyone who chose to continue by phone. At first I didn't know how long I would continue this monthly commute, but promised to do it for at least a year. Toward the end of that year I came to the further decision that, in order to continue to provide viable analytic treatment to this group of phone-therapy patients, a number of whom were still in prolonged "regressions to dependence," I needed to commit to coming to see them once a month *indefinitely*. This, I realize, was an unusual, possibly unique, choice on my part. It grew out of my particular analytic values and way of being an analyst. It also worked for me in that it allowed me to actively maintain my closest Chicago friendships, and later, as it happened, to see my daughter once a month during her entire four years of college—facts that all of my patients were aware of.

The two patients from whose treatments the following notes were drawn are both in this group. The first, Simone, had been in once-a-week analytic therapy for about two years prior to my move; the second, Mary, had been in what I consider twice-a-week analysis for about the same length of time. These sessions took place in Chicago during one of my regular visits, about a year and a half after I had begun the monthly schedule. Thus, at the time of the sessions, both had been in treatment with me for about five years.

Simone

Simone, a woman in her 60s, is a sister in a small but well-regarded international Catholic order that has one of its largest communities in Chicago. She has many talents, both interpersonally and in a business sense, that make her valuable to her community. She is very bright and competent in an unpretentious way, unusually empathic and supportive in her relationships, and a natural leader with good political instincts; thus many sisters in her community are drawn to her and depend on her for help and support of one kind or another. Simone's problem is that it is very hard for her to say no, set limits, or assert herself when too much is asked of her, when another sister is not pulling her own weight, or worst of all, if she is being threatened, undermined or attacked by someone who is competitive with her or has ambitions of her own.

During the five years of work leading up to the following session, Simone and I have worked at this issue from many angles. We have come to understand her deep need to be loved, accepted, and valued; her extreme discomfort with conflict and confrontation; her moral commitment to being there for those who need her; and her moral aversion to anyone who exhibits a sense of selfish entitlement. We recognize that both her moral commitments and personality organization have their roots in her childhood, during which, from an early age, she understood that she had to be very grown up and help her father deal with her schizophrenic mother. She does not feel conscious resentment about this. She views her father as a good and loving man in a difficult situation, and doesn't begrudge him his need for her assistance. At the same time, she is aware that she carries a painful loneliness just under the surface, and pays a significant price for not being more assertive when she should be. She becomes overextended, cranky, and has a moderate eating disorder wherein she eats too many unhealthy foods—clearly a compensation for feeling emotionally depleted. Many of our sessions are spent exploring her experience in situations where she feels resentful but can't bring herself to assert herself.

Notes from April 15 session

R has missed work at the hospice for three weeks. [R is a sister who lives with Simone who rarely pulls her own weight around the house or in the community, incurring the resentment of many. Simone is critical and resentful too, but is far more comfortable complaining to me about it than saying anything to R.] *Has to talk to E about the New York house. Thinking of bringing up their relationship. Feeling more comfortable with this.* [E is the current "provincial" or head of Simone's community in America and oversees all community business (a position Simone had held in the past). Among Simone's many talents, she understands real estate, and has been entrusted by the community to sell an extremely valuable property owned by the order in New York City. Yet E has opposed Simone on certain aspects of the sale of this property, which annoys Simone, hurts her feelings, and creates tension between them that is hard for Simone to tolerate. E is someone whom Simone has felt intermittently hurt by and alienated from during the past few years. They had once been close friends, but when E became provincial she became more distant and critical with Simone. It was the tensions in this relationship that had originally prompted Simone to seek therapy with me. She has spent many of our sessions talking about this, and has, with my help, come to view E's unfriendliness as coming more from E's problems—especially her feeling threatened by Simone, who is more competent than E in many ways.]

At some point I said her community was lucky to have her—a member who had so many competencies. How would they deal with some of these problems without her? She talked about feeling more confidence and less vulnerability vis-à-vis E. Feeling better and not sure why. This was posed as a question to me. I wondered whether anything stood out in the recent period of our work. She mentioned work we had done in relation to her mother—her loneliness as a child. But also work on present things with E. I agreed: it was probably a "cycling through" the stuff with her mother, the stuff with E, and a deepening in our relationship [she had recently acknowledged for the first time her awareness of her dependency on me]. *At this point she said she felt very held by me in our relationship. Felt a sense of peace. Knows I really care about her and understand her experience—what she feels. She trusts me. It's a very good feeling.*

Commentary

Among the many intersubjective facts bearing on Simore's experience in this session, we certainly would have to consider first the fact that we were meeting in person—a relative rarity. I would say it is true of all of my Chicago patients that they feel more psychologically held during our in-person sessions, and that the experience of being held stands out in a different way than if we were in person all the time. Yet, Simone and I had been meeting in person on a monthly basis for a year and a half prior to this session, and this was the first time she made reference to peaceful feelings; so clearly more was involved.

I would say that Simone and I have had an "easier" relationship in that there has always been a good rapport. I enjoy her and genuinely respect her values and competencies. It is also clear that she enjoys, respects, and appreciates me as her therapist. She is one of a number of patients who have given me an inside view of the Catholic world, which I find both fascinating and disturbing. She is high functioning not just in her level of achievement and capacity to function in the world, but in her psychological/emotional development. In many ways, she enjoys life. This allows for a certain ease in our relationship. Humor has played a part in our relationship, though not in the present session. Parenthetically, I would say that humor itself can be conducive to at least momentary experiences of analytic peace, and can function cumulatively in an analytic relationship as one intersubjective factor leading to the achievement of analytic peace in a deeper sense. I might say that all of these factors between Simone and me create a kind of envelope of relative peace in our relationship. This alone does not constitute or account for the experience of analytic peace that she reports in this session. But I believe the emotional tone of an analytic relationship can certainly be a contributing factor to the achievement of analytic peace.

Truly, I cannot know what accounts for Simone's experience of peace. It is too complex, really infinitely complex, and the secret is hopelessly "locked" in her subjectivity, to which I will never have access. My best guess is that there was a convergence of factors. One was the work she and I had done over years regarding her relationship with E. The derailments with E had been a continuing source of pain, anxiety and stress. We had revisited the problem many times, and it now seemed she truly felt she was making progress with it. Part of my understanding of her progress is that I had come to feel increasingly confident in my hypotheses about the causes of E's treatment of Simone, and had been expressing them with greater certainty, even a cavalier authoritativeness. I think my confidence was beginning to convince her that E's treatment of her had little to do with her—or at least with anything she had done "wrong"—and was emboldening her to deal with E from a position of greater self-confidence.

I also think our recent opening up, in a new way, the exploration of her emotional life as a child, especially in relation to her mother, had made possible, or at least held the promise of, a new level of integration. In identifying her *early* profound loneliness as an implicit or unconscious factor driving her *current* adaptation, and sensitizing her to any possible loss or rejection, not only did Simone have a new, useful understanding with which she resonated, it had also deepened and consolidated something in our connection as a working, analytic team. It signified that I could see her child-self, was empathic to that self, and was interested in incorporating the "voice" of that child-self into our exploratory dialogue. This development had to be part of what she meant by saying she felt "very held." Indeed, I'm sure this development was part of what allowed her to acknowledge feeling more dependent, which acknowledgment itself represented a deepening engagement with me. There was also the practical sense in which these new insights afforded us greater leverage in analyzing future experiences either with E, or with others. We had understood for a long time that there was a transference element in her relationship with E, and now we had a deeper understanding of it. For example, I had been able to make the recent interpretation that since E had become provincial, E's experience of, and behavior toward, Simone had a crazy quality to it, perhaps unconsciously signaling that Simone had lost E as she had lost her mother to schizophrenia.

The only other factor I am aware might have contributed to Simone's experience that day was my general "analytic mood." I think that, for reasons unknown, I was feeling some sense of peace, or readiness to engage, or "on-ness" that infused all that I did and said, and that this may have increased my general acuity, my capacity to hold, and at the same time been somewhat contagious. In this sense, although Simone's experience of peace was multi-determined, it may, in this particular session, have started in me.

Mary

I have written about Mary at an earlier point in our work (S. Stern, 2007; Chapter 7 in this volume). Now in her mid-50s, Mary has settled into her twice-a-week analysis in a deep way, having worked through anxieties described in the earlier write-up.

One aspect of our early work was her concern, during approximately the first year and a half, that I was not sufficiently warm or actively affirming to help her with her relentlessly self-attacking inner voice—the voice of her primitively intrusive, controlling, critical, guilt-and-shame-inducing mother with whom she had identified (S. Stern, 2002a, b, 2007). These anxieties had led to an enactment in which I felt increasingly deficient as a therapist and person, wishing I could be different than I was, and thinking that perhaps Mary would be better off with a different therapist. When it finally occurred to me that I was feeling something very similar to what she had been made to feel as a child, and still felt, I had an "outburst" (Mitchell, 1997) in which I made this interpretation while at the same time asserting that I could only be the person I was, that I would try to be as affirming as I could, but that I had limitations that we would both have to live with. In retrospect, seen through the theoretical lens I have been developing in the present chapter, this was an instance in which Mary's struggle came powerfully into the transference-countertransference dynamic, precipitating an inner struggle on my part, leading to my emotionally charged, heart-felt intervention. The result was a necessary grieving process for both of us (which I believe lies at the heart of the resolution of many such enactments), and ultimately the intersubjective achievement of a greater sense of acceptance and peace with each other. This peace has been a lasting one. In the wake of my outburst, and Mary's and my processing of it, Mary settled into our relationship in a new way, and that sense of commitment has deepened over time.

Mary's response to my decision to leave Chicago was unique and impressive: she consciously resolved to use the time in between my announced decision and my final move (when I would no longer be commuting weekly and seeing her in person every session) to try to accomplish as much as she could. What she and I both quickly realized was that this meant she would be seeking to deepen her engagement with me just as I was leaving! She grasped the possible defensive element in this, but she and I both sensed that this was not the fundamental meaning of her resolution. The deeper meaning was that she had already chosen me as the person with whom she wanted to try to work through her struggle to feel more psychically alive, and she was determined to fully engage that struggle despite my geographic relocation.

True to her resolution, our relationship did deepen significantly during the two years between my announcement and final move. One dimension of this process was a period of months when Mary became almost psychotically depressed during our sessions. She remained (barely) able to function well-enough outside of sessions, but in my presence she felt so anxious that, in her experience of it, she was literally unable to think. She felt unbearably depressed but claimed to have no understanding, or even clue, about what was causing the depression. We, of course, explored the likely possibility that it related to my leaving, but this exploration led nowhere; the depression really did not seem to be about that. Thus, we were both totally stymied for what seemed an endless period. She consulted with her psychiatrist who, for the first time, put her on a low dose of an anti-psychotic medication in addition to her anti-depressant. This helped a little with her functioning outside of sessions, but had no effect on her in-session experience.

It is hard to describe what these sessions were like. Mary would sit across from me, essentially mute for most of the time, but acutely anxious because she felt her inability to say more about her state reflected a profound inadequacy on her part. Moreover, the anxiety circled around on itself in that her anxiety about not being able to articulate anything interfered with her ability to think in a comfortably reflective way, making her feel empty-headed, totally helpless, hopeless, and worried to the point of panic that I would lose patience with her—in fact, was already silently feeling fed up with her psychological ineptitude.

I became aware of a growing paradoxical tension in me. On the one hand, I felt it was important to "stay with" whatever was happening in Mary, with no hint of expectation that she need do anything to resolve her own tension as far as I was concerned. If she felt too anxious to think, we would stay with her anxiety and see what emerged. In accord with this part of my thinking, I simply remained silent with her throughout many sessions, sincerely feeling that this was the kind of holding environment she needed. On the other hand, it became increasingly clear that Mary was not going to be able to think her way through this—her capacity for reflective self-awareness was too disabled by her anxiety. I was somehow going to have to help her figure out her depression relying only on my own reverie process and powers of inference (Ogden, 1994, 1997). This paradoxical understanding and stance is another example of what I mean by *contouring* (see Chapter 3).

At some point I began to consider the possibility that Mary's depression had something to do with her upcoming annual visit home at Thanksgiving. These visits had always been significant events in Mary's life, and in the analysis, because of the psychic damage they inevitably wrought. Usually, we spent considerable session time both anticipating, and helping her recover from, these visits. The reason I didn't make the connection this time was because Mary didn't either. Usually, she was all too aware of her anticipatory anxiety, and totally devastated in the aftermath, such that we spent much time talking about it all. But this time there was no conscious anticipatory anxiety, only Mary's mute depression. I started thinking about this conundrum and realized that, during the past year since her last visit, Mary, with my help, had finally confronted the fact that her older sister, who had functioned as a substitute mother for her as a young child and early adolescent, had not really functioned in that role since the sister had left for college many years ago. Mary had maintained a powerful, mostly unconscious, maternal transference to her for all these years, despite messages from the sister, who was now married with her own children, that she no longer wished to function in this way. In fact, she had become critical and devaluing of Mary, much like Mary's real mother. Mary had finally seen the truth of her sister's repudiation of the maternal role, and it now occurred to me that her seemingly inexplicable depression was a profound and prolonged grieving process (or melancholic aborting of such a process) for the loss of the person whom she had thought of as her mother.

When I made this interpretation, tentatively, it was as if a dam broke. She sobbed deeply and resonated in such a profound way that it seemed clear she was not just responding to suggestion. Beginning immediately, she experienced enormous relief that her depression actually had meaning. There was also a sense of gratitude that I had survived her depression and anxiety without losing patience, and had been able to supply the capacity to think about her experience that had been submerged in her anxiety. Also, starting immediately, she began to be able to think and speak in the sessions, and the period of mute depression was replaced by her usual, more animated, participation.

As will become evident shortly, I review all this in part to provide the background regarding the meaning, in Mary's analysis, of her capacity/incapacity to think, and to give a feel for the temporal dimension of the analytic process leading to experiences of analytic peace. The sessions described in the following notes took place approximately two and a half years following this dark period in Mary's treatment and about a year and a half following my final move to Maine.

Notes from April 15 session

Powerful session. Her dream of losing Jeero and looking for him in a department store like the department store of her childhood and past dreams. There is a special gift offer of Jeeros. She's angry. I interpret that this symbol of her good self/world/object is taken over by her mother's world.

[Jeero is one of a series of small stuffed animals ("Ugly Dolls") that Mary collects. Jeero is a favorite, and she had given me one as a goodbye gift when I had moved a year and a half earlier. I have my Jeero on my desk in my Maine office, which she knows. Mary had had many stuffed animals and puppets as a child, creating a whole fantasy world into which she escaped and spent much time. Most of these creatures were benign and friendly, creating a good world that contrasted sharply with the threatening, crazy world that she actually inhabited.

Department stores were the setting of many highly aversive scenes from Mary's childhood, all involving her mother. Her mother would take her clothes shopping, always trying to dress Mary according to the mother's image of how she should look, and always critically commenting on defects in Mary's body or the way she looked in clothes that did not meet with the mother's approval. Also, the mother herself was a pathological shopper, buying many things that she subsequently returned because the desired object became a defective object once she possessed it.]

I interpret that she evacuated all her good self into her stuffed animals and puppets. They were empathic, kind, thoughtful, comforting, and alive. Meanwhile, she took in all the bad from her mother—which colonized, and still occupies, her.

Videoconferencing. [We had, at her urging, been contemplating trying this for our phone sessions.] *Ambivalent: the camera objectifies her—she'll look small and pathetic. Her mother's demeaning characterization of her, and John (her husband): "He's a small man." I comment on her sensitivity to her sense of whether or not I see her (including her physical self) as good.*

She brought up her evanescent, tearful emotions. [She had been telling me for some time of episodes when, seemingly unbidden and mysteriously, she found herself feeling like crying or actually becoming tearful. These episodes signified to both of us some kind of coming to life—a thawing of buried, frozen, painful feelings of unclear origin and meaning.] *Most of these episodes occur when she's not here* [in session], *in between things. She wants to cry here more fully but can't. I wonder out loud: "Would the sadness be too much? Would the emotions be too painful to tolerate?" At this point she remembers our last session before I moved—boxes all around. She could cry, but felt peaceful with me. She remembers telling me to be quiet when I over-talked. Something about my presence, the way I listen, the way I am with her, makes her feel peaceful.*

She becomes tearful. We sit quietly with this for a while. Finally I say: It's her thinking that's the problem. When she thinks on her own, she thinks herself into a bad place—always! With me, in my presence, this now moderates. She can, at times, think more freely, and begin to feel things other than anxiety. In between sessions, her affects come up in between things, when she's not *thinking. As soon as she stops thinking, her feelings emerge. She likes this and agrees.*

[At the end of the note I have an afterthought, which I jot down.]

Peace—Analytic Peace. Peace as an intersubjective co-creation.

Commentary

A number of strands of our work are coming together in this session. The background reality, always, for Mary is her relentless self-excoriation, which, to say the least, precludes any experience of inner peace. The question, from the beginning of our work together, has been whether I will be able to help her think and feel differently about herself. She knows that I understand this, and is hopeful that I can help. The long period of inexplicable depression before my move illustrates just how bad this can get. She had shown me her most disabled self, placing herself completely in my hands, which represented a deepening dependency even as I was about to leave. Fortunately, we did work through this: I had been able to hold her in her most paralyzing state of anxiety and depression, and in the end had been able to think for her, resulting in the resumption of her (still-compromised) ability to think. Thus, by the time of my actual move—that unspeakably sad day when we sat surrounded by my boxes—she could experience her grief, yet, at the same time, a sense of peace being in my presence. She had had to tell me to be quiet: *she*, apparently, feeling more at peace than I was. She didn't want me interfering with her grieving.

I had known about her stuffed animal collection for a long time. Not only had she had this as a child, she still had one now, as an adult. I had understood previously that her stuffed animals were crucial to her survival as a child. Recently, I had understood further and interpreted that they represented a form of creativity that was part of her core self. It seemed remarkable to me that she had created this world of beings, which were clearly not transitional objects in Winnicott's sense because they did not represent her mother (or at least her actual mother), but were entirely of her own creation. Jeero, as he functioned in our relationship was perhaps her first true transitional object. I had further emphasized that this created world indicated that a part of her was, in fact, alive, even though she otherwise felt dead. The theme of Mary's latent creativity had become an increasing focus in our work, and she had recently had a dream in which she was figure skating in a very free and graceful way, signifying to her a release of her creative potential. Now, in this session, I have the further thought and interpret that, for reasons we don't yet understand, she projected all the good in her onto these stuffed fantasy creatures while she herself took in all the bad her mother projected into her, and experienced nothing else.

This leads back to her actual current state of mind, wherein, significantly, there are beginning to be cracks in her deadening inner narrative, and signs of life—moments of inexplicable tearfulness—popping up through the cracks. I am able to see more clearly than ever before the pervasive, destructive, unstoppable nature of her negative thinking, and the fact that our cumulative work to this point is beginning to create a breach in her inner monologue. Mostly, she still needs to be in my presence (which can include phone as well as in-person sessions) to experience this breach, and the relief (peace) that comes with it. But now she is beginning to experience brief openings in between sessions, and I interpret that these seem to be occurring in between things: i.e., when she's not thinking about herself or the business of her life.

In short, our work and my presence are creating moments of peace, alongside intimations of life, which include both the possibility of greater freedom and creativity (no longer just projected into her puppets), and the emergence of yet-unspeakable pain. These gains, however, are highly precarious, and could, at any moment, be confiscated or reabsorbed back into the department store world of her mother.

I have to ask myself: Why did the idea of analytic peace emerge for me after this session with Mary? Of course, I can't really know. I think I was feeling a sense of awe at the complex interpenetration of her psyche and mine—the complexity of our particular version of progressive intersubjective fittedness. And I think *I* was feeling a form of relative peace as the session evolved—aware that our close work was helping her feel more peaceful and alive. I think I must have been (at least unconsciously or preconsciously) very aware of the two-way nature of our interchange. Sometimes, it was me who helped her find peace, but sometimes it was the other way around, as during the last session before my move. Finally, it seems in retrospect, that creativity was in the air. We were talking about the survival value of her latent creativity, and somehow our dialogue simultaneously prompted a creative impulse on my part—an enactment of the ever-mysterious co-creative dialogue of analysis.

Conclusion

Analytic peace is an elusive concept, as elusive as the processes through which it is attained. From a certain perspective one might wonder whether the concept is substantial enough to warrant as much attention as I have given it. Almost by definition, successful psychotherapy brings with it a greater sense of peace, usually for both parties. So, what is the gain from naming and focusing on it, particularly if, as I have said, seeking to achieve it may work against actually doing so?

My personal answer is that to have the concept in mind provides a kind of balance to our work—a balance that, in and of itself, constitutes a deepening of analytic wisdom. We are very aware of the reality of struggle—in our patients' lives and in our analytic work. We understand now, better than at any previous point in our profession's history, that analytic work, by definition, entails struggle. Contemporary psychoanalytic theory has awakened us to the fact that the struggle is always—indeed, must become—intersubjective if the patient's struggles are to be fully engaged and addressed. It is the back and forth, dialectical movement between the subjective and the intersubjective experience of these struggles to which the analyst must attend (Benjamin, 1990; Ogden, 1994; Stolorow, 1997b). Even as we understand the centrality of struggle, it is helpful to keep in mind that the transformation or resolution of analytic struggle is synonymous with the emergence of analytic peace. Struggle and peace in psychoanalysis, as in life, exist in essential dialectical tension. Applying Ogden's (1986) definition of a dialectical relationship: struggle and peace "create, inform, preserve, and negate each other" (p. 208). Given this core underlying tension and structure, it seems important to be cognizant of both poles of this dialectic that so fundamentally defines our work.

Beyond this basic existential grounding, I believe having peace in mind as a deeply implicit analytic aim orients us in subtle, visceral ways to where the immediate analytic work of the moment—the patient's current struggle—resides. And although we don't usually set out to directly transform the patient's state of struggle into one of peace, having peace in mind informs our approach to entering, sensing, mapping, and engaging the patient's experiential world and struggles in increasingly fitted ways. As I hope both the theoretical arguments and clinical vignettes in this chapter, and throughout this book, have demonstrated, such an orientation yields interventions that ultimately move the dyad and patient *through struggle* toward experiences of relative peace, which, in both their meaning and character, are unique to that dyad and that patient.

Appendix

The forward edge of the relational unconscious: a theoretical comparison

The Boston Change Process Study Group (BCPSG) (2013), Grossmark (2012a, b), and Aron and Atlas (2015) have each offered models of a forward-tending dimension of the relational unconscious. Each has areas of overlap, but also certain differences, with the model I propose in Chapter 4 of an intersubjective-systemic tendency toward progressive relational fittedness in analytic dyads. It is useful to briefly clarify those similarities and differences.

The Boston Change Process Study Group (BCPSG) (2013)

The Boston Change Process Study Group (2013) finds a forward-tending movement toward increasing systemic complexity and competence to be a characteristic of implicit relational processes in analytic dyads, evidenced most dramatically during enactments. They argue that enactments, rather than being a manifestation of dissociated traumatic relational experience from the patient's past, as Relationalists have theorized, represent the emergence ("eruption") of new, more complex and therapeutically potent modes of interaction that had already begun to occur implicitly as part of the dyad's natural movement toward greater complexity and fittedness.

Given that their thinking is significantly influenced by Sander's (2008) ideas about mother-infant and analytic dyads as complex systems, there is significant overlap in our approaches. I agree, for example, that what I am calling the forward edge of the relational unconscious tends to move toward greater complexity and relational fittedness. But they seem to be arguing that *all* enactments:

> . . . signal that a new sense of possibility is emerging or has emerged, a potential openness in the dyad to change in the old pattern of relating. This eruption of something new into the process further opens the possibility of the dyad's finding new ways of being together.
>
> (2013, p. 737)

This very optimistic perspective seems useful as a *hypothesis* to hold in mind as a possible understanding of *some* enactments, or certain dimensions of enactments. But, as a general theory of enactments, I question it on two major grounds.

First, it seems to me an example of the error of *mistaking the part for the whole* addressed in Chapter 1. Following from the principles of uniqueness and specificity espoused throughout this book, I don't believe there is any single dynamic that accounts for all enactments. Thus, I agree with the BCPSG that there is a forward edge dimension of the relational unconscious, or, to use their language, of the "implicit relationship." And I believe that all enactments can usefully be understood *in relation to* this implicit forward tendency. But exactly how they relate is unique to each situation. Plus, it seems intuitively more plausible that many enactments represent, at least in part, *derailments* of the movement toward greater complexity and fittedness.

My second disagreement concerns their apparent view of the dyad's unconscious movement toward progressive complexity, competence and fittedness as an *automatic* property of the dyad as a dynamic system. While they don't exactly state this, it is a necessary corollary of their view of enactments as always emanating from this movement toward new ways of being together. While I believe there is always a forward edge dimension to *the patient's* implicit participation, including during enactments, I don't think the same is necessarily true of enactments themselves. In a sense, we could say that it is the patient's "job" to enact—something we have known ever since Freud (1912a) recognized the existence and centrality of transference. But, as I have emphasized in different contexts throughout the previous chapters, the fate of a given interaction, especially enactments, in relation to the dyad's movement toward greater fittedness and complexity, is hardly automatic, but rather depends on the analyst's capacities to *meet* the patient "in the enactment" in ways that move toward greater specificity of recognition and connection. Unlike the more natural, automatic, forward developmental tendency of good enough parents and their infants, such forward movement in an analytic couple cannot be assumed, but rather relies on the analyst's highly evolved, complex grasp of the situation, or at least of his approach to *trying* to grasp the situation, in order for "simply human," needed interactions to emerge. Perhaps the BCPSG wrote their paper with this as an unstated assumption. But, I would argue that, *even if* the analyst can be assumed to have the necessary evolved sensibility, this still is no guarantee that a given enactment will resolve in the direction of greater fittedness and productive complexity.

Grossmark (2012a, b)

Without naming it as such, Grossmark has proposed a theory of enactments with an implied forward edge dimension of unconscious engagement. He also emphasizes the importance of "meeting" patients in the space of enactment. But his vision of the necessary kind of meeting is somewhat different than mine; thus comparing the two approaches is instructive.

His theory begins with the intriguing proposal that, rather than seeking to detect and interpret the problematic or defensive meanings of enactments in an effort to transform or "get out of" them, analysts would do better to regard and treat them as the relational equivalent of free association. In a spirit akin to Bion's (1970) seeking "at-one-ment with O," Grossmark suggests that analysts "unobtrusively" seek to enter "the flow of enactive engagement," trusting that flow to carry both patient and analyst into the vortex of the patient's unmetabolized trauma and generate interactive processes that enable a reworking and transformation of the patient's underlying traumatized states and relational needs. Thus, not unlike Bion, Grossmark is advocating a paradoxical stance of intending to participate in the unintentional, and thereby changes the meaning and *nature* of the unintentional.

Grossmark's model connects directly with the central themes of this book. He is suggesting that we do better to trust the patient's unconscious motivations and participation to evoke the kinds of analyst participation that the patient most needs. He thereby similarly converts the hermeneutic of suspicion usually associated with Relational approaches to enactments to a hermeneutic of trust, and, within that context, posits that, if the analyst can allow himself "unobtrusively" to fit in with the patient's relational needs and idiom of engagement, the co-created, unconscious relationship will spontaneously tend toward certain kinds of emergent fittedness. Also very much in the integrative spirit of this book, Grossmark (2012b), in constructing his model, "borrows from various threads of the contemporary psychoanalytic tapestry, including relational, object relations, contemporary Freudian, British Independent, self psychology, intersubjective, infant research and more" (p. 630).

The point on which he and I may diverge is the generality of his concept of "the unobtrusive relational analyst." Grossmark (2012a, b) develops and presents this concept in the context of his work with two patients with similar relational needs. Although very different people, both patients seemed to require a high level of control over the analyst's participation, and a non-interpretive, non-interventionist analyst who allowed himself to work responsively within the patient's relational idiom. This approach indeed seemed to be transformative in both of these cases; but then Grossmark proceeds to advocate this stance as a general participatory model for relational analysts. If this is his intention, I believe he also makes the error of *mistaking the part for the whole* discussed in the Introduction. While I agree with his intention (following M. Balint [1968] and E. Balint [1993]) of meeting or "accompanying" each patient within his or her unique idiom of relational need, it is hardly the case that all or even most analytic patients, including many primitively organized patients, need their analyst to be exclusively unobtrusive in the way Grossmark describes.

For example, in the first treatment I briefly summarized in Chapter 1, while the patient needed me to be unobtrusive in Grossmark's sense for several years, in the later phases of the analysis she needed the opposite: for me to be much more interactive and personally forthcoming. The progression in that case was along the lines Slochower (1996) has theorized: The patient initially required a holding environment with little intrusion from my subjectivity; but then, with greater consolidation in her sense of self, shifted into a mode of needing and *wanting* my more "real" subjective participation. Shane, Shane, and Gales (1997) and Teicholz (1999), have written about similar progressions.

My work with Sam also calls Grossmark's assumptions into question. Had I simply, "unobtrusively," continued go with the flow of enactive engagement indefinitely, I believe, given Sam's underlying passivity and dissociative character defense, that he and I would have remained stuck in our directionless coupled oscillator. I wouldn't characterize my ultimate interventions with Sam as trying either to interpret or get out of our partially enactive state. Rather, acting on my intuitive sense of unease, I made "expressive use of my countertransference" (Bollas, 1987) in a way that *opened up* our enactive dynamic to collaborative processing and a different kind of relational flow, which, in my view, was needed in the service of Sam's unconscious developmental struggles and aims.

I find Grossmark's contribution especially generative, and believe that the deceptively simple frame of reference he is aiming for has wide applicability with many, perhaps in some sense with all, of our patients. The idea of fitting in with the patient's idiom of needed relationship, of meeting patients in their spontaneous process and allowing oneself to be, in a sense, carried along by that process, even in the turbulent waters of what we call enactments, and through periods of concern, doubt, and uncertainty, is a radical idea that turns the concept of enactment on its head. In a sense, I have been advocating something similar in the idea of "meeting patients in spaces where being met is an alien, distrusted experience" (Chapter 1, p. 28). The difference is that I don't equate entering "the flow of enactive engagement" with being "unobtrusive" in the way that Grossmark describes his participation in his two cases. These patients needed him to be unobtrusive, but other patients have very different relational needs with their analysts. In my work with Linda, presented in both Chapters 1 and 6, I see myself as having entered a flow of enactive engagement with her; but that relational flow involved me in a complexly paradoxical stance of simultaneously accepting and confronting her defenses against attachment, commitment and dependency. I believe Linda, in effect, asked me to do this very thing in our first session: "I need someone to hold my feet to the fire." I'm not sure if Grossmark would view my response to this desperate request as obtrusive or unobtrusive within his scheme.

If this is indeed a real difference, then I would reassert my preference for the terms "needed relationship," "meeting," "fittedness," and "specificity of recognition and connection" as the more generalizable language—generalizable because it is completely non-prescriptive and assumes that "the flow of enactive engagement" will take unique, fluid forms in every case.

Aron and Atlas (2015)

Aron and Atlas (2015) have recently offered a rich synthesis and creative extension of various trends in psychoanalytic thought, beginning with

Jung (1912), all focusing on a forward-looking dimension and function of the unconscious. Departing from Freud's predominant interest in the determining unconscious influence of the past on present experience, Jung found a "prospective function" contained in symbols and dreams—an active, teleological dimension of the unconscious which pulls us toward our destiny, and anticipates, rehearses, constructs, and shapes future possibilities. The authors join Grossmark (2012a), the BCPSG (2013), myself (S. Stern 1994), and other relational theorists (broadly defined) by extending Jung's ideas to the area of analytic interaction and enactments. Unlike Grossmark and the BCPSG, and more similar to my (1994) thinking, they view enactments as having both a prospective and a repetitive dimension; or, to use Tolpin's (2002) terms, both a "forward edge" and a "trailing edge." This is different from Grossmark's and the BCPSG's formulations in that the latter authors, as I have just reviewed, propose reframing enactments as *fully* prospective when interpreted and/or managed in light of the theoretical schemes they are advocating.

At the same time, Aron and Atlas' formulation is similar to Grossmark's and the BCPSG's, and different than mine, in that they argue that their prospective dimension is "generative and transformative in and of itself": that is, they view many enactments as having an inherently forward-looking dimension—an unconscious fitting together—that serves a therapeutically transformative function, sometimes for both parties. While I can agree that this may be the case in certain instances, this is a somewhat different conceptualization than my view of the forward edge of the relational unconscious as synonymous with an intersubjective tendency toward progressive fittedness. While I believe the systemic tendency toward fittedness assumes a shared motivation to move in that direction, such movement is usually far from automatic: It requires effort and work, especially on the part of the analyst. Thus, while *reaching* for fittedness may be an inherent property of the system, *achieving* it is not.

Bibliography

Alizade, M. (2010). *Psychoanalysis and positivity.* London: Karnac.

Anderson, J.W. (2005). The psychobiographical study of psychologists. In W.T. Shultz, (Ed.), *Handbook of psychobiography* (pp. 203–209). New York: Oxford University Press.

Aron, L. (1996). *A meeting of minds: Mutuality in psychoanalysis.* Hillsdale, NJ: The Analytic Press.

Aron, L. (2006). Analytic impasse and the third: Clinical implications of intersubjectivity theory. *International Journal of Psychoanalysis*, *87*: 349–368.

Aron, L. (2009). Day, night, or dawn: Commentary on paper by Steven Stern. *Psychoanalytic Dialogues*, *19*: 656–668.

Aron, L. (2012). The current state of relational psychoanalysis: Polarization, thirds, pluralism, eclecticism, and integration. Paper presented at the 33rd Annual Spring Meeting of Division 39 (Psychoanalysis) of the American Psychological Association, Boston, MA, April 24–28.

Aron, L. & Starr, K. (2013). *A psychotherapy for the people: Toward a progressive psychoanalysis.* New York and London: Routledge.

Aron, L. & Atlas, G. (2015). Generative enactment: Memories from the future. *Psychoanalytic Dialogues*, *25*: 309–324.

Atwood, G.E. & Stolorow, R.D. (1984). *Structures of subjectivity.* Hillsdale, NJ: The Analytic Press.

Bacal, H.A. (1998). *Optimal responsiveness: How therapists heal their patients.* Northvale, NJ: Jason Aronson.

Bacal, H.A. (2011). *The power of specificity in psychotherapy: When therapy works and when it doesn't.* Plymouth, UK: Jason Aronson.

Bach, S. (2006). *Getting from here to there: Analytic love and analytic process.* Hillsdale, NJ: The Analytic Press.

Bakhtin, M.M. (1981). *The dialogic imagination: Four essays. (M. Holquist, Ed. & Trans.).* Austin, TX: University of Texas Press.

Balint, E. (1993). *Before I was I: Psychoanalysis and the imagination.* London: Guilford.

Balint, M. (1968). *The basic fault.* London: Tavistock.

Baranger, M. & Baranger, W. (1961–1962/2009). The analytic situation as a dynamic field. *International Journal of Psychoanalysis, 89*: 795–826.

Baruch, H. (2014). The compass for psychoanalytic action: Discussion of Steven Stern's "Analytic adoption of the psychically homeless." Paper presented at the Annual Conference of the International Association for Psychoanalytic Self Psychology, Jerusalem, Oct. 21–25, 2014.

Bass, A. (2007). When the frame doesn't fit the picture. *Psychoanalytic Dialogues, 17*: 1–27.

Bass, A. (2015). The dialogue of unconsciouses, mutual analysis and the uses of the self in contemporary relational psychoanalysis. *Psychoanalytic Dialogues, 25*: 2–17.

Bateman, A.W. & Fonagy, P. (2016). *Mentalization-based treatment for personality disorders: A practical guide.* Oxford, UK: Oxford University Press.

Beebe, B. (2004). Symposium on intersubjectivity in infant research and its implications for adult treatment. IV. Faces-in-relation: A case study. *Psychoanalytic Dialogues, 14*: 1–51.

Beebe, B. & Lachmann, F.M. (2002). *Infant research and adult treatment: Co-constructing interactions.* Hillsdale, NJ: The Analytic Press.

Beebe, B. & Lachmann, F.M. (2014). *The origins of attachment: Infant research and adult treatment.* London: Routledge.

Benjamin, J. (1988). *The bonds of love: Psychoanalysis, feminism, and the problem of domination.* New York: Pantheon.

Benjamin, J. (1990). Recognition and destruction: An outline of intersubjectivity. *Psychoanalytic Psychology, 7*(suppl.): 33–47.

Benjamin, J. (2002). The rhythm of recognition: Comments on the work of Louis Sander. *Psychoanalytic Dialogues, 12*: 43–54.

Benjamin, J. (2004). Beyond doer and done to: An intersubjective view of thirdness. *Psychoanalytic Quarterly, 73*: 5–46.

Bion, W.R. (1959). *Experiences in groups and other papers.* New York: Basic Books.

Bion, W.R. (1962). *Learning from experience.* In *Seven Servants.* New York: Aronson, 1977.

Bion, W.R. (1965). *Transformations.* New York: Basic Books.

Bion, W.R. (1967). Notes on memory and desire. In J. Aguayo and B. Malin (Eds.), *Wilfred Bion: Los Angeles seminars and supervision* (pp. 136–138). London: Karnac, 2013.

Bion, W.R. (1970). *Attention and interpretation.* London: Karnac.

Bion, W.R. (1987). *Clinical seminars and other works.* London: Karnac, 2000.

Bollas, C. (1987). *Shadow of the object: Psychoanalysis of the unthought known.* New York: Columbia University Press.

Bollas, C. (1989). *Forces of destiny: Psychoanalysis and human idiom*. Northvale, NJ: Jason Aronson.

Boston Change Process Study Group (2008). Forms of relational meaning: Issues in the relations between the implicit and reflective-verbal domains. *Psychoanalytic Dialogues, 18*: 125–148.

Boston Change Process Study Group (2010). *Change in psychotherapy: A unifying paradigm*. New York: W.W. Norton.

Boston Change Process Study Group (2013). Enactment and the emergence of new relational organization. *Journal of the American Psychoanalytic Association, 61*: 727–749.

Bowlby, J. (1975). *Attachment and loss, Vol. 1*. New York: Basic Books.

Bowlby, J. (1988). *A secure base: Clinical applications of attachment theory*. London: Routledge.

Brandchaft, B. (1994). To free the spirit from its cell. In R.D. Stolorow, G.E. Atwood, & B. Brandchaft (Eds.), *The intersubjective perspective* (pp. 57–76). Northvale, NJ: Jason Aronson.

Brandchaft, B. (2010). Toward an emancipatory psychoanalysis. In B. Brandchaft, S. Doctors, & D. Sorter, *Toward an emancipatory psychoanalysis: Brandchaft's intersubjective vision* (pp. 9–27). New York and London: Routledge.

Brandchaft, B., Doctors, S., & Sorter, D. (2010). *Toward an emancipatory psychoanalysis: Brandchaft's intersubjective vision*. New York and London: Routledge.

Bromberg, P.M. (1989). Interpersonal psychoanalysis and self psychology: A clinical comparison. In *Standing in the spaces: Essays on clinical process, trauma, and dissociation* (pp. 147–162). Hillsdale, NJ: The Analytic Press, 1998.

Bromberg, P.M. (1991). On knowing one's patient inside out. *Psychoanalytic Dialogues, 1*: 399–422.

Bromberg, P.M. (1998). *Standing in the spaces: Essays on clinical process, trauma, and dissociation*. Hillsdale, NJ: The Analytic Press.

Bromberg, P.M. (2006). *Awakening the dreamer: Clinical journeys*. Mahwah, NJ: The Analytic Press.

Bromberg, P.M. (2011). *The shadow of the tsunami and the growth of the relational mind*. New York and London: Routledge.

Brothers, D. (2008). *Toward a psychology of uncertainty: Trauma-centered psychoanalysis*. New York and London: Routledge.

Coburn, W.J. (2002). A world of systems: The role of systemic patterns of experience in the therapeutic process. *Psychoanalytic Inquiry, 22*: 655–677.

Coburn, W.J. (2014). *Psychoanalytic complexity: Clinical attitudes for therapeutic change*. New York and London: Routledge, Kindle Edition.

Cooper, S. (2014). The things we carry: Finding/creating the object and the analyst's self-reflective participation. *Psychoanalytic Dialogues, 24*: 621–636.

Corpt, E. (2011). Clinical generosity: An attitude deeply embedded in contemporary self psychology. Paper presented at the Annual Conference, International Association for Psychoanalytic Self Psychology. Los Angeles, CA.

Damasio, A. (1994). *Descartes' error: Emotion, reason, and the human brain.* New York: Penguin.

Damasio, A. (1999). *The feeling of what happens: Body and emotion in the making of consciousness.* New York: Harcourt.

Davies, J.M. (1994). Love in the afternoon: A relational consideration of desire and dread in the countertransference. *Psychoanalytic Dialogues, 4*: 153–170.

Davies, J.M. (2004). Whose bad object are we anyway? Repetition and our elusive love affair with evil. *Psychoanalytic Dialogues, 14*: 711–732.

Davies, J.M. & Frawley, M.G. (1994). *Treating the adult survivor of childhood sexual abuse.* New York: Basic Books.

Eigen, M. (1981). The area of faith in Winnicott, Lacan, and Bion. *International Journal of Psycho-Analysis, 62*: 413–433.

Eigen, M. (1996). *Psychic deadness.* Northvale, NJ: Jason Aronson.

Ehrenberg, D.B. (1992). *The intimate edge: Extending the reach of psychoanalytic interaction.* New York: W.W. Norton.

Fairbairn, W.R.D. (1952). *Psychoanalytic studies of the personality.* London: Tavistock.

Fairbairn, W.R.D. (1958). On the nature and aims of psychoanalytic treatment. *International Journal of Psycho-Analysis, 39*: 374–383.

Ferenczi, S. (1915). Psychogenic anomalies of voice production. In J. Richman (Ed.), *Further contributions to the theory and technique of psychoanalysis* (pp. 105–109). London: Karnac, 1980.

Ferenczi, S. (1928). The elasticity of psycho-analytic technique. In M. Balint (Ed.), *Final contributions to the problems and methods of psycho-analysis* (pp. 87–101). London: Karnac, 1980.

Ferenczi, S. (1933). Confusion of tongues between adults and the child. In M. Balint (Ed.), *Final contributions to the problems and methods of psycho-analysis* (pp. 156–167). London: Karnac, 1980.

Ferro, A. (2005). *Seeds of illness, seeds of recovery: The genesis of suffering and the role of psychoanalysis.* London: Routledge.

Ferro, A. & Basile, R. (2009). *The analytic field: A clinical concept.* London: Karnac.

Ferro, A. & Civitarese, G. (2013). Analysts in search of an author: Voltaire or Artemisia Gentileschi? Commentary on "Field theory in psychoanalysis, part 2:

Bioinian field theory and contemporary interpersonal/relational psychoanalysis." *Psychoanalytic Dialogues, 23*: 646–653.

Ferro, A. & Civitarese, G. (2015). Confrontation in the Bionian model of the analytic field. Chapter 7 in *The analytic field and its transformations*. London: Karnac (Kindle Edition).

Fonagy, P. (2001). *Attachment theory and psychoanalysis.* New York: Other Press.

Fonagy, P., Gergely, G., Jurist, E.L., & Target, M. (2002). *Affect regulation, mentalization, and the development of the self.* New York: Other Press.

Fosshage, J.L. (2003). Contextualizing self psychology and relational psychoanalysis: Bi-directional influence and proposed syntheses. *Contemporary Psychoanalysis, 39*: 411–448.

Fosshage, J.L. (2007). Searching for love and expecting rejection: Implicit and explicit dimensions in cocreating analytic change. *Psychoanalytic Inquiry, 27*: 326–347.

Frankel, J.B. (1993). Collusion and intimacy in the analytic relationship: Ferenczi's legacy. In L. Aron & A. Harris (Eds.), *The Legacy of Sandor Ferenczi* (pp. 227–247). Hillsdale, NJ: Analytic Press.

Freud, A. (1937). *The ego and the mechanisms of defense.* London: Hogarth Press.

Freud, A. (1954). The widening scope of indications for psychoanalysis: Discussion. *Journal of the American Psychoanalytic Association, 2*: 607–620.

Freud, S. (1912a). The dynamics of transference. In J. Strachey (Ed. & Trans.), *The standard edition of the complete psychological works of Sigmund Freud* (Vol. 12, pp. 99–120). London: Hogarth Press, 1958.

Freud, S. (1912b). Recommendations to physicians practicing psycho-analysis. In J. Strachey (Ed. & Trans.), *The standard edition of the complete psychological works of Sigmund Freud* (Vol. 12, pp. 111–120). London: Hogarth Press, 1958.

Freud, S. (1913). On beginning the treatment. In J. Strachey (Ed. & Trans.), *The standard edition of the complete psychological works of Sigmund Freud* (*Vol. 12*, pp. 123–144). London: Hogarth Press, 1958.

Freud, S. (1914). Remembering, repeating, and working through. In J. Strachey (Ed. & Trans.), *The standard edition of the complete psychological works of Sigmund Freud* (*Vol. 12*, pp. 147–156). London: Hogarth Press, 1958.

Freud, S. (1915a). Observations on transference-love. In J. Strachey (Ed. &Trans.), *The standard edition of the complete psychological works of Sigmund Freud* (Vol. 12, pp. 159–171). London: Hogarth Press, 1958.

Freud, S. (1915b). The unconscious. In J. Strachey (Ed. & Trans.), *The standard edition of the complete psychological works of Sigmund Freud* (Vol. 14, pp. 166–215). London: Hogarth Press, 1957.

Freud, S. (1917). Mourning and melancholia. In J. Strachey (Ed & Trans.), *The standard edition of the complete psychological works of Sigmund Freud* (Vol. 14, pp. 243–258). London: Hogarth Press, 1957.

Freud, S. (1926). Inhibitions, symptoms and anxiety. In J. Strachey (Ed. & Trans.), *The standard edition of the complete psychological works of Sigmund Freud* (Vol. 20, pp. 77–175). London: Hogarth Press, 1959.

Freud, S. (1940). An outline of psychoanalysis. In J. Strachey (Ed. & Trans.), *The standard edition of the complete psychological works of Sigmund Freud* (Vol. 23, pp. 141–207). London: Hogarth Press, 1964.

Gabbard, G.O. & Ogden, T.H. (2009). On becoming a psychoanalyst. *International Journal of Psychoanalysis*, *90*: 311–327.

Gadamer, H.-G. (1965). *Truth and method.* G. Barden & J. Cumming (Trans.). London: Continuum, 2004.

Galatzer-Levy, R. (1978). Qualitative change from quantitative change: Mathematical catastrophe theory in relation to psychoanalysis. *Journal of the American Psychoanalytic Association*, *26*: 921–935.

Galatzer-Levy, R. (2002). Emergence. *Psychoanalytic Inquiry*, *22*: 708–727.

Galatzer-Levy, R. (2009). Good vibrations: Analytic process as coupled oscillations. *International Journal of Psychoanalysis*, *90*: 983–1007.

Gardner, R.M. (1983). *Self-inquiry.* Boston and Toronto: Little, Brown and Company.

Gedo, John E. (1979). *Beyond interpretation*: *Toward a revised theory for psychoanalysis.* New York: International Universities Press.

Gedo, J.E. & Goldberg, A. (1973). *Models of the mind.* Chicago: University of Chicago Press.

Geist, R.A. (2007). Who are you, who am I, and where are we going: Sustained empathic immersion in the opening phase of psychoanalytic treatment. *International Journal of Psychoanalytic Self Psychology*, *2*: 1–26.

Geist, R.A. (2009). Empathy, connectedness, and the evolution of boundaries in self psychological treatment. *International Journal of Psychoanalytic Self Psychology*, *4*: 165–180.

Gerson, S. (2004). The relational unconscious: A core element of intersubjectivity, thirdness, and clinical process. *Psychoanalytic Quarterly*, *73*: 63–98.

Gerson, S. (2009). When the third is dead: Memory, mourning, and witnessing in the aftermath of the holocaust. *International Journal of Psychoanalysis*, *90*: 1341–1357.

Ghent, E. (1990). Masochism, submission, surrender: Masochism as a perversion of surrender. *Contemporary Psychoanalysis*, *26*: 108–136.

Ghent, E. (2002). Wish, need, drive: Motive in light of dynamic systems theory and Edelman's selectionist theory. *Psychoanalytic Dialogues*, *12*: 763–808.

Gill, M.M. (1979). The analysis of the transference. *Journal of the American Psychoanalytic Association*, *27*: 263–288.

Gill, M.M. (1982). *Analysis of transference, Vol. 1.* New York: International Universities Press.

Gill, M.M. (1994). *Psychoanalysis in transition: A personal view.* Hillsdale, NJ: The Analytic Press.

Gill, M.M. & Hoffman, I.Z. (1982). *Analysis of transference, Vol. 2.* New York: International Universities Press.

Goldberg, A. (1999). *Being of two minds: The vertical split in psychoanalysis and psychotherapy.* Hillsdale, NJ: Analytic Press.

Goldstein, J. (2007). Emergence and psychological morphogenesis. In C. Piers, J. P. Muller & J. Brent (Eds.), *Self-organizing complexity in psychological systems* (pp. 156–167). New York: Jason Aronson.

Green, A. (1975). The analyst, symbolization, and absence in the analytic setting (On changes in analytic practice and analytic experience). *International Journal of Psycho-Analysis*, *43*: 436–440.

Greenberg, J. & Mitchell, S. (1983). *Object relations in psychoanalytic theory.* Cambridge, MA: Harvard University Press.

Greenson, R.R. (1967). *The technique and practice of psychoanalysis.* New York: International Universities Press.

Grossmark, R. (2012a). The flow of enactive engagement. *Contemporary Psychoanalysis*, *48*: 287–300.

Grossmark, R. (2012b). The unobtrusive relational analyst. *Psychoanalytic Dialogues*, *22*: 629–646.

Harris, A. (2004). The relational unconscious: Commentary on papers by Michael Eigen and James Grotstein. *Psychoanalytic Dialogues*, *14*: 131–137.

Harris, A. (2005). *Gender as soft assembly.* Hillsdale, NJ: The Analytic Press.

Harris, A. (2009). "You must remember this." *Psychoanalytic Dialogues*, *19*: 2–21.

Harris, A. & Aron, L. (1997). Ferenczi's semiotic theory: Previews of postmodernism. *Psychoanalytic Inquiry*, *17*: 522–534.

Havens, L. (1989). *A safe place: Laying the groundwork of psychotherapy.* Cambridge, MA: Harvard University Press.

Hoffman, I.Z. (1983). The patient as interpreter of the analyst's experience. *Contemporary Psychoanalysis*, *19*: 389–422.

Hoffman, I.Z. (1992). Expressive participation and psychoanalytic discipline. *Contemporary Psychoanalysis*, *28*: 1–15.

Hoffman, I.Z. (1994). Dialectical thinking and therapeutic action. *Psychoanalytic Quarterly*, *63*: 187–218.

Hoffman, I.Z. (1998). *Ritual and spontaneity in the psychoanalytic process: A dialectical-constructivist view.* Hillsdale, NJ: The Analytic Press.

Hoffman, I.Z. (2009). Therapeutic passion in the countertransference. *Psychoanalytic Dialogues, 19*: 617–637.

IARPP Colloquium Series: No. 28, May 9–May 22, 2016.

James, W. (1908). *Talks to teachers of psychology; and to students on some of life's ideals*. New York: Henry Holt.

Joseph, B. (1989). *Psychic equilibrium and psychic change: Selected papers of Betty Joseph.* (M. Feldman & E.B. Spillius, Eds.) London: Routledge.

Jung, C. G. (1912). *Psychology of the unconscious: A study of the transformations and symbolisms of the libido, a contribution to the history of the evolution of thought* (B.M. Hinkle, trans., 1916; rev. 1952 as Symbols of transformation, selected works, Vol. 5), London, UK: Kegan, Paul, Trench, Trubner.

Kainer, R.G.K. (1999). *The collapse of the self and its therapeutic restoration.* Hillsdale, NJ: Analytic Press.

Keats, J. (1817/1952). Letter to George and Thomas Keats, 21 December, 1817. In *Letters* ed. by M.B. Forman. 4th Edition. London: Oxford University Press.

Klein, M. (1946). Notes on some schizoid mechanisms. In *Envy and gratitude and other works, 1946–1963* (pp. 1–24). New York: Delacorte, 1975.

Knoblauch, S.H. (2000). *The musical edge of therapeutic dialogue.* Hillsdalé, NJ: The Analytic Press.

Kohut, H. (1959). Introspection, empathy, and psychoanalysis. *Journal of the American Psychoanalytic Association, 7*: 459–483.

Kohut, H. (1971). *The analysis of the self: A systematic approach to the psychoanalytic treatment of narcissistic personality disorders.* New York: International Universities Press.

Kohut, H. (1977). *The restoration of the self.* New York: International Universities Press.

Kohut, H. (1982). Introspection, empathy, and the semicircle of mental health. *International Journal of Psychoanalysis, 63*: 395–408.

Kohut, H. (1984). *How does analysis cure?* (A. Goldberg & P. Stepansky, Eds.) Chicago: University of Chicago Press.

Krystal, H. (1988). *Integration and self-healing: Affect, trauma and alexithymia.* Hillsdale, NJ: Analytic Press.

Lacan, J. (1977). *Ecrits: A selection.* New York: W.W. Norton.

Lakoff, G. & Johnson, M. (1980). *Metaphors we live by.* Chicago: University of Chicago Press.

Lakoff, G. & Johnson, M. (1999). *Philosophy in the flesh.* New York: Basic Books.

LeDoux, J. (2009). Why the "right brain" idea is wrong-headed. *The Huffington Post.* Retrieved from http://www.huffingtonpost.com/joseph-ledoux/why-the-right-brain-idea_b_206156.html.

Levenson, E.A. (1972). *The fallacy of understanding.* New York: Basic Books.

Levenson, E.A. (1983). *The ambiguity of change: An inquiry into the nature of psychoanalytic reality.* New York: Basic Books.

Levinas, E. (1969). *Totality and infinity: An essay on externality.* Pittsburgh, PA: Duquesne University Press.

Lipton, S.D. (1977). The advantages of Freud's technique as shown in his analysis of the Rat Man. *International Journal of Psychoanalysis, 58*: 255–273.

Loewald, H. (1960). On the therapeutic action of psychoanalysis. In *Papers on Psychoanalysis* (pp. 221–256). New Haven: Yale University Press, 1980.

Loewald, H. (1979). Reflections on the psychoanalytic process and its therapeutic potential. In *Papers on Psychoanalysis* (pp. 372–383). New Haven: Yale University Press, 1980.

Loewald, H. (1980). *Papers on psychoanalysis.* New Haven: Yale University Press.

Lynn, D.J. & Valliant, G.E. (1998). Anonymity, neutrality, and confidentiality in the actual methods of Sigmund Freud: A review of 43 cases, 1907–1939. *American Journal of Psychiatry, 155*: 163–171.

Lyons-Ruth, K. (1999). The two-person unconscious: Intersubjective dialogue, enactive relational representation, and the emergence of new forms of relational organization. *Psychoanalytic Inquiry, 19*: 576–617.

Lyons-Ruth, K. (2000). "I sense that you sense that I sense": Sander's recognition process and the specificity of relational moves in the psychotherapeutic setting. *Journal of Infant Mental Health, 21*: 85–99.

Lyons-Ruth, K., Bruschweiler-Stern, N., Harrison, A.M., Morgan, A.C., Nahum, J.P., Sander, L.W., & Tronick, E.Z. (1998). Implicit relational knowing: Its role in development and psychoanalytic treatment. *Infant Mental Health Journal, 19*: 282–289.

Lyons-Ruth, K. & Jacobvitz, D. (2008). Attachment disorganization, genetic factors, parenting contexts, and developmental transformation from infancy to adulthood. In J. Cassidy & P. Shaver (Eds.), *Handbook of attachment: Theory, research, and clinical applications, second edition* (pp. 666–698). New York: Guilford.

Marks-Tarlow, T. (2008). *Psyche's veil: Psychotherapy, fractals and complexity.* London and New York: Routledge.

Marks-Tarlow, T. (2011). Merging and emerging: A non-linear portrait of intersubjectivity during psychotherapy. *Psychoanalytic Dialogues, 21*: 110–127.

McDougall, J. (2001). The psychic economy of addiction. In J. Petrucelli & C. Stuart (Eds.), *Hungers and compulsions: The psychodynamic treatment of eating disorders and addictions* (pp. 3–26). Northvale, NJ: Jason Aronson.

McLaughlin, J. (1991). Clinical and theoretical aspects of enactment. *Journal of the American Psychoanalytic Association, 39*: 595–614.

Mendelsohn, E. (2007). Analytic love: Possibilities and limitations. *Psychoanalytic Inquiry, 27*: 219–245.

Mitchell, S.A. (1988). *Relational concepts in psychoanalysis: An integration.* Cambridge, MA: Harvard University Press.
Mitchell, S.A. (1993). *Hope and dread in psychoanalysis.* New York: Basic Books.
Mitchell, S.A. (1997). *Influence and autonomy in psychoanalysis.* Hillsdale, NJ: The Analytic Press.
Mitchell, S.A. (2000). *Relationality.* Hillsdale, NJ: The Analytic Press.
Modell, A.H. (1993). *The private self.* Cambridge, MA: Harvard University Press.
Neri, C. (2009). The enlarged notion of field in psychoanalysis. In A. Ferro and R. Basile (Eds.), *The analytic field: A clinical concept.* London: Karnac.
Nhat Hanh, T. (1998). *The heart of the Buddha's teaching: Transforming suffering into peace, joy, & liberation.* Berkeley, CA: Parallax Press.
Ogden, T.H. (1986). *The matrix of the mind: Object relations and the psychoanalytic dialogue.* Northvale, NJ: Jason Aronson.
Ogden, T.H. (1994). *Subjects of analysis.* Northvale, NJ: Jason Aronson.
Ogden, T.H. (1997). *Reverie and interpretation: Sensing something human.* Northvale, NJ: Jason Aronson.
Ogden, T.H. (1999). "The music of what happens" in poetry and psychoanalysis. *International Journal of Psychoanalysis, 80*: 979–994.
Ogden, T.H. (2004). An introduction to the reading of Bion. *International Journal of Psycho-analysis, 85*: 285–300.
Ogden, T.H. (2005). *The art of psychoanalysis.* London and New York: Routledge.
Ogden, T.H. (2009). *Rediscovering psychoanalysis.* London and New York: Routledge.
Ogden, T.H. (2015). Intuiting the truth of what's happening: On Bion's "Notes on Memory and Desire." *Psychoanalytic Quarterly, 84*: 285–306.
Ogden, T.H. & Gabbard, G.O. (2010). The lure of the symptom in psychoanalytic treatment. *Journal of the American Psychoanalytic Association, 58*: 533–544.
Orange, D.M. (1995). *Emotional understanding: Studies in psychoanalytic epistemology.* New York: Guilford.
Orange, D.M. (2002). There is no outside: Empathy and authenticity in psychoanalytic process. *Psychoanalytic Psychology, 19*: 686–700.
Orange, D.M. (2008). Recognition as: Intersubjective vulnerability in the psychoanalytic dialogue. *International Journal of Psychoanalytic Self Psychology, 3*: 178–194.
Orange, D.M. (2011). *The suffering stranger.* New York and London: Routledge.
Orange, D.M. (2012). Development and response to the other: Engagement and Enactment as bridging concepts among contemporary psychoanalytic groups. Ottawa, St. Paul University, April 20, 2012.
Orange, D.M. (2014). And we shall be changed: To hold theory lightly is to surrender assumptions: Discussion of clinical narrative by Steven Stern. *International Journal of Psychoanalytic Self Psychology, 9*: 193–199.

Peltz, R. (2012). Ways of hearing: Getting inside psychoanalysis. *Psychoanalytic Dialogues*, *22*: 279–290.

Peltz, R. & Goldberg, P. (2013). Field conditions: Discussion of Donnel B. Stern's "Field theory and psychoanalysis." *Psychoanalytic Dialogues*, *23*: 660–666.

Petrucelli, J. & Stuart, C. (Eds.). (2011). *Hungers and compulsions: The psychodynamic treatment of eating disorders & addictions.* Northvale, NJ: Jason Aronson.

Pizer, S.A. (1998). *Building bridges: The negotiation of paradox in psychoanalysis.* Hillsdale, NJ: The Analytic Press.

Pizer, S.A. (2004). Impasse recollected in tranquility: Love, dissociation, and discipline in the analytic process. *Psychoanalytic Dialogues*, *14*: 289–311.

Pizer, S.A. (2014). The analyst's generous involvement: Recognition and the "tension of tenderness." *Psychoanalytic Dialogues*, *22*: 1–13.

Poland, W.S. (2000). The analyst's witnessing and otherness. *Journal of the American Psychoanalytic Association*, *48*: 17–34.

Racker, H. (1968). *Transference and countertransference.* New York: International Universities Press.

Reich, W. (1933). *Character analysis.* New York: Farrar, Straus and Giroux, 1949.

Reis, B. (2009). Performative and enactive features of psychoanalytic witnessing: The transference as the scene of address. *International Journal of Psychoanalysis. 90*: 1359–1372.

Reis, B. (2011). Silence and quiet: A phenomenology of wordlessness. Panel presentation at the annual spring meeting of the American Psychological Association, Division 39, New York, NY.

Renik, O. (1993). Analytic interaction: Conceptualizing technique in light of the analyst's irreducible subjectivity. *The Psychoanalytic Quarterly*, *62*: 553–571.

Renik, O. (2006). Practical *psychoanalysis for therapists and patients.* New York, NY: Other Press.

Ricoeur, P. (1970). *Freud and philosophy: An essay on interpretation.* New Haven, CT: Yale University Press.

Ringstrom, P.A. (1998). Therapeutic impasses in contemporary psychoanalytic treatment: Revisiting the double bind hypothesis. *Psychoanalytic Dialogues*, *8*: 297–316.

Ringstrom, P. (2001). Cultivating the improvisational in psychoanalytic treatment. *Psychoanalytic Dialogues*, *11*: 727–754.

Ringstrom, P. (2007). Scenes that write themselves: Improvisational moments in relational psychoanalysis. *Psychoanalytic Dialogues*, *17*: 69–99.

Rozmarin, E. (2009). I am yourself: Subjectivity and the collective. *Psychoanalytic Dialogues*, *19*: 604–616.

Russell, P.L. (1998). Trauma and the cognitive function of affects. In J.G. Teicholz & D. Kriegman (Eds.), *Trauma, repetition, and affect regulation: The work of Paul Russel* (pp. 23–47). New York: The Other Press.

Russell, P.L. (2006). The theory of the crunch. In *Smith College Studies in Social Work, Volume 26*. Haworth Press, 9–21.

Rustin, J. & Sakaer, C. (2004). From the neuroscience of memory to psychoanalytic interaction. *Psychoanalytic Psychology*, *21*: 70–82.

Sander, L. (1995). Identity and the experience of specificity in a process of recognition: Commentary on Seligman and Shanok. *Psychoanalytic Dialogues*, *5*: 579–592.

Sander, L. (2002). Thinking differently: Principles of process in living systems and the specificity of being known. *Psychoanalytic Dialogues*, *12*: 11–42.

Sander, L. (2008). *Living systems, evolving consciousness, and the emerging person: A selection of papers from the life work of Louis Sander* (G. Amadei & I. Bianchi, Eds.). New York and London: Routledge.

Sandler, J. (1960). The background of safety. *International Journal of Psychoanalysis*, *41*: 352–356.

Schaefer, R. (1983). *The analytic attitude.* New York: Basic Books.

Schore, A.N. (1994). *Affect regulation and origin of the self: The neurobiology of emotional development.* Hillsdale, NJ: Lawrence Erbaum Associates.

Schore, A.N. (2003). *Affect regulation and the repair of the self.* New York: W.W. Norton.

Schore, A.N. (2011). Foreword. In *The shadow of the tsunami and the growth of the relational mind* by P.M. Bromberg. New York and London: Routledge, pp. ix–xxxvi.

Schwaber, E. (1983). Psychoanalytic listening and psychic reality. *International Review of Psychoanalysis*, *10*: 379–392.

Seligman, S. (2005). Dynamic systems theories as a metaframework for psychoanalysis. *Psychoanalytic Dialogues 15*: 285–319.

Shane, E. (2006). Developmental systems self psychology. *International Journal of Psychoanalytic Self Psychology*, *1*: 23–45.

Shane, M., Shane, E., & Gales, M. (1997). *Intimate attachments: Toward a new self-psychology.* New York: Guilford.

Shaw, D. (2014). *Traumatic narcissism: Relational systems of subjugation.* New York: Routledge.

Slade, A. (2014). Imagining fear: Attachment, threat, and psychic experience. *Psychoanalytic Dialogues*, *24*: 253–266.

Slavin, J.H. (2007). The imprisonment and liberation of love: The dangers and possibilities of love in the psychoanalytic relationship. *Psychoanalytic Inquiry*, *27*: 197–218.

Slavin, M.O. (2010). On recognizing the psychoanalytic perspective of the other: A discussion of "Recognition as: Intersubjective vulnerability in the psychoanalytic dialogue" by Donna Orange. *International Journal of Psychoanalytic Self Psychology*, *5*: 274–292.

Slavin, M.O. & Kriegman, D. (1992). *The adaptive design of the human psyche: Psychoanalysis, evolutionary biology, and the therapeutic process.* New York: The Guilford Press.

Slavin, M.O. & Kriegman, D. (1998). Why the analyst needs to change: Toward a theory of conflict, negotiation, and mutual influence in the therapeutic process. *Psychoanalytic Dialogues*, *8*: 247–284.

Slochower, J. (1996). Holding and the fate of the analyst's subjectivity. *Psychoanalytic Dialogues*, *6*: 323–353.

Stern, D.N., Sander, L.W., Nahum, J.P., Harrison, A.M., Lyons-Ruth, K., Morgan, A.C., Bruschweiler-Stern, N., & Tronick, E.Z. (1998). Non-interpretive mechanisms in psychoanalytic therapy: The "something more" than interpretation. *International Journal of Psychoanalysis*, *79*: 903–921.

Stern, D.B. (1990). Courting surprise: Unbidden perceptions in clinical practice. *Contemporary Psychoanalysis*, *26*: 452–478.

Stern, D.B. (2003). The fusion of horizons: Dissociation, enactment, and understanding. *Psychoanalytic Dialogues*, *13*: 843–873.

Stern, D.B. (2010). *Partners in thought: Working with unformulated experience, dissociation, and enactment.* New York and London: Routledge.

Stern, D.B. (2013a). Field theory in psychoanalysis, part 2: Bionian field theory and contemporary interpersonal/relational psychoanalysis. *Psychoanalytic Dialogues*, *23*: 630–645.

Stern, D.B. (2013b). Responses to commentaries by Ferro and Civitarese, Carnochan, Peltz and Goldberg, and Levine. *Psychoanalytic Dialogues*, *23*: 674–682.

Stern, D.B. (2013c). Relational freedom and therapeutic action. *Journal of the American Psychoanalytic Association*, *61*: 227–255.

Stern, S. (1992). The opposing currents technique: For eating disorders and other false self problems. *Contemporary Psychoanalysis*, 28: 594–615.

Stern, S. (1994). Needed relationships and repeated relationships: An integrated relational perspective. *Psychoanalytic Dialogues*, *4*: 317–346

Stern, S. (2002a). The self as a relational structure: A dialogue with multiple-self theory. *Psychoanalytic Dialogues*, *12*: 693–714.

Stern, S. (2002b). Identification, repetition, and psychological growth: An expansion of relational theory. *Psychoanalytic Psychology*, *19*: 722–738.

Stern, S. (2004). The yin and yang of intersubjectivity: Integrating self-psychological and relational thinking. *Progress in Self Psychology*, *20*: *Transformations in Self Psychology*. Hillsdale, NJ: The Analytic Press.

Stern, S. (2007). The conundrum of self-care. *Contemporary Psychoanalysis*, *43*: 605–620.

Stern, S. (2008). In praise of language. *International Journal of Psychoanalytic Self Psychology*, *3*: 504–506.

Stern, S. (2009a). Session frequency and the definition of psychoanalysis. *Psychoanalytic Dialogues, 19*: 639–655.

Stern, S. (2009b). What's possible? What matters? Reply to commentaries. *Psychoanalytic Dialogues, 19*: 691–703.

Stern, S. (2009c). The dialectic of empathy and freedom. *International Journal of Psychoanalytic Self Psychology, 4*: 132–164.

Stern, S. (2011). The therapeutic action of analytic love: Commentary on Joye Weisel-Barth's "Katherine: A long hard case." *International Journal of Psychoanalytic Self Psychology, 6*: 489–504.

Stern, S. (2014a). A 9-year analysis with a connection-resistant patient: Theory, reality and the messiness of therapeutic action. *International Journal of Psychoanalytic Self Psychology, 9*: 179–192.

Stern, S. (2014b). Finding a language of shared power: Reply to Donna Orange and David Wallin. *International Journal of Psychoanalytic Self Psychology, 9*: 208–216.

Stern, S. (2015). Identification vs. dissociation: A needed dialectic between two "principles of mental functioning." Paper presented at the 12th Annual Conference of the International Association for Relational Psychoanalysis and Psychotherapy, Toronto, Ontario, June 25–28, 2015.

Stern, S. (In preparation). *The airless world: A relational metapsychology of disabled selves.* Book in preparation.

Stolorow, R.D. (1994). The nature of the therapeutic action of psychoanalytic interpretation. In R.D. Stolorow, G.E. Atwood, & B. Brandchaft (Eds.), *The intersubjective perspective* (pp. 43–55). Northvale, NJ: Jason Aronson.

Stolorow, R.D. (1997a). Dynamic, dyadic, intersubjective systems: An evolving paradigm for psychoanalysis. *Psychoanalytic Psychology, 14*: 337–364.

Stolorow, R.D. (1997b). Principles of dynamic systems, intersubjectivity, and the obsolete distinction between one-person and two-person psychologies. *Psychoanalytic Dialogues, 7*: 859–868.

Stolorow, R.D. (2006). Autobiographical and theoretical reflections on the "ontological unconscious." *Contemporary Psychoanalysis, 42*: 233–241.

Stolorow, R.D. (2014). Undergoing the situation: Emotional dwelling I is more that empathic understanding. *International Journal of Psychoanalytic Self Psychology, 9*: 80–83.

Stolorow, R.D. & Atwood, G.E. (1979). *Faces in a cloud: Subjectivity in personality theory.* Northvale, NJ: Jason Aronson.

Stolorow, R.D. & Atwood, G.E. (1992). *Contexts of being.* Hillsdale, NJ: The Analytic Press.

Stolorow, R.D., Atwood, G.E., & Brandchaft, B. (1994) (Eds.). *The intersubjective perspective.* Northvale, NJ: Jason Aronson.

Stolorow, R.D., Atwood, G.E., & Orange, D.M. (2002). *Worlds of experience: Interweaving philosophical and clinical dimensions in psychoanalysis.* New York: Basic Books.

Stolorow, R.D., Brandchaft, B., & Atwood, G.E. (1987). *Psychoanalytic treatment: An intersubjective approach.* Hillsdale, NJ: The Analytic Press.

Stolorow, R.D., Orange, D.M., & Atwood, G.E. (1998). Projective identification begone!: Commentary on paper by Susan H. Sands. *Psychoanalytic Dialogues, 8*: 719–725.

Stone, L. (1954). The widening scope of indications for psychoanalysis. *Journal of the American Psychoanalytic Association, 2*: 567–594.

Strachey, J. (1934). The nature of the therapeutic action of psychoanalysis. *International Journal of Psycho-Analysis, 44*: 432–443.

Sullivan, H.S. (1953). *The interpersonal theory of psychiatry.* New York: Norton.

Sullivan, H.S. (1954). *The psychiatric interview.* New York: Norton.

Symington, N. (1983). The analyst's act of freedom as agent of therapeutic change. *International Review of Psychoanalysis, 10*: 283–292.

Symington, N. (2012). The essence of psycho-analysis as opposed to what is secondary. *Psychoanalytic Dialogues, 22*: 395–409.

Tansey, M.J. & Burke, W.F. (1989). *Understanding countertransference.* Hillsdale, NJ: The Analytic Press

Teicholz, J.G. (1999). *Kohut, Loewald, and the postmoderns: A comparative study of self and relationship.* Hillsdale, NJ: The Analytic Press.

Teicholz, J.G. (2000). The analyst's empathy, subjectivity, and authenticity: Affect as the common denominator. In *How Responsive Should We Be: Progress in Self Psychology, 16*. Hillsdale, NJ: The Analytic Press, 33–53.

Teicholz, J.G. (2002). Some further thoughts on the analyst's empathy and authenticity. Presented at Institute for Contemporary Psychoanalysis, Los Angeles, February 3, 2002.

Teicholz, J.G. (2006). Qualities of engagement and the analyst's theory. *International Journal of Psychoanalytic Self Psychology, 1*: 47–77.

Teicholz, J.G. (2015). Blurring the boundaries between contemporary psychoanalytic theories: Does the new research bring an end to our old beloved distinctions? Paper presented at the 38th Annual Conference of the International Association of Psychoanalytic Self Psychology, Oct. 15–18, Los Angeles, CA.

Thelen, E. (2005). Dynamic systems theory and the complexity of change. *Psychoanalytic Dialogues, 15*: 255–283.

Thelen, E. & Smith, L. (1994). *A dynamic systems approach to the development of cognition and action.* Cambridge, MA: MIT Press.

Tolpin, M. (2002). Doing psychoanalysis of normal development: Forward edge transferences. *Progress in Self Psychology, 18*: 167–190.

Tronick, E. (1998). Dyadically expanded states of consciousness and the process of therapeutic change. *Infant Mental Health Journal, 19*: 290–299.

Tronick, E. (2007). *The neurobehavioral and social-emotional development of infants and children.* New York: W.W. Norton.

VanDerHeide, N. (2007). Authenticity and psychoanalytic technique: A reconsideration. *International Journal of Psychoanalytic Self Psychology, 2*: 275–289.

Wachtel, P.L. (2014). When the context is in the room: Extending the relational paradigm. *Psychoanalytic Dialogues, 24*: 419–426.

Waddell, M. (2002). *Inside lives: Psychoanalysis and the growth of the personality.* London: Karnac.

Wallin, D. (2007). *Attachment and psychotherapy.* New York: Guilford.

Wallin, D. (2014). Because connection takes two: The analyst's psychology in treating the "connection-resistant" patient. *International Journal of Psychoanalytic Self Psychology, 9*: 200–207.

Weisel-Barth, J. (2011). Katherine: A long hard case. *International Journal of Psychoanalytic Self Psychology, 6*: 444–468.

Weiss, P. (1970). Whither life science? *American Scientist, 58*: 156–163.

Weiss, J., Sampson, H., & the Mount Zion Psychotherapy Research Group (1986). *The psychoanalytic process: Theory, clinical observations and empirical research.* New York: Guildford Press.

Winnicott, C. (1978). D.W. Winnicott: A reflection. In S. Grolnick, L. Barkin & W. Muensterberger (Eds.), *Between reality and fantasy.* New York: Jason Aronson.

Winnicott, D.W. (1949). Hate in the countertransference. *International Journal of Psycho-Analysis, 30*: 69–75.

Winnicott, D.W. (1954). Metapsychological and clinical aspects of regression within the psycho-analytical set-up. In *Through Pediatrics to Psychoanalysis* (pp. 278–294). New York: Basic Books, 1975.

Winnicott, D.W. (1956). Primary maternal preoccupation. In *Through pediatrics to psycho-analysis* (pp. 300–305). New York: Basic Books, 1975.

Winnicott, D.W. (1960a). The theory of the parent-infant relationship. In *The Maturational Processes and the Facilitating Environment* (pp. 37–55). New York: International Universities Press, 1965.

Winnicott, D.W. (1960b). Ego distortion in terms of true and false self. In *The maturational processes and the facilitating environment* (pp. 140–152). New York: International Universities Press.

Winnicott, D.W. (1962). The aims of psycho-analytic treatment. In *The Maturational Processes and the Facilitating Environment* (pp. 166–178). New York: International Universities Press, 1965.

Winnicott, D.W. (1965). *The maturational processes and the facilitating environment.* New York: International Universities Press.
Winnicott, D.W. (1969). The use of an object and relating through identifications. In *Playing and Reality* (pp. 86–94). London: Tavistock Publications.
Winnicott, D.W. (1971a). *Playing and Reality.* London: Tavistock Publications.
Winnicott, D.W. (1971b). *Therapeutic consultations in child psychiatry.* London: Karnac.

Index